ERRONEOUS PSYCHIATRIC SELF-DIAGNOSIS

:

Non-Psychiatric Patients that Present at a Psychiatrist's Office

:

[WITH EXTENSIVE BIBLIOGRAPHIES]

Robert Charles Powell, MD, PhD

North Charleston, SC:
CreateSpace Independent Publishing Platform, 2015
Copyright © 2015
Robert Charles Powell

ISBN-10:1512322571
ISBN-13: 9781512322576

First Edition: May 2015
10 9 8 7 6 5 4 3 2 1

[censored manuscript][1]

---

[1] The owner of the medical facility where these patients were evaluated refused to allow publication of any specific medical data, lest this reflect negatively on the non-psychiatric units of the facility.

Part of the problem was that some of the ignored lab results were so astoundingly aberrant as to render patient confidentiality close to impossible. The censored items in these "brief case reports" generally included age, presenting complaint, relevant parts of the elicited recent past mental status, past medical history (including use or not of medications, alcohol, nicotine, vitamins, and minerals), and lab results.

The focus of the uncensored version of the manuscript had been on demonstrating that frequently the initial clinical histories along with the past lab values were sufficient to suggest probable non-neuropsychiatric conditions, which then could be confirmed by judiciously chosen lab tests. Specialty lab tests were NOT ordered on every patient.

Obviously, publishing the raw data would be best, but presenting the argument without the censored data still should raise a few questions – and a few alarms. Of 750 patients presenting for initial psychiatric evaluation, over one-third were found to have previously undiagnosed non-neuropsychiatric conditions. In the original manuscript only the worst half of these cases was presented.

"It often falls on neuropsychiatrists to recognize conditions which ... do not belong to their particular field of inquiry, yet which have a definite bearing on the neuropsychiatric evaluation of the ... total organism."

Paul I. Yakovlev

"the appropriate response to a test requires going beyond just noting that a result is outside the range of normal ... ."

Ilse R. Wiechers, Felicia A. Smith, Theodore A. Stern

I. Iron Deficiency (especially in men)

> "It is widely held that iron-deficiency anemia, not associated with organic disease, is rare in adolescent or adult male subjects ...." W Brumfitt

An amazing number of patients – especially young males – present with the erroneous psychiatric self-diagnosis of "anxiety" or "depression" when iron deficiency is more likely the primary problem. Recognizing this has been impeded by the continuing general assumption that iron deficiency is primarily a problem faced by women of childbearing age – that is, certainly not by otherwise healthy young men – although accumulating data suggest otherwise. First let me present several of the most illustrative cases seen in an outpatient psychiatric practice over the last three years; overall, about six per cent of the newly evaluated patients were found to have iron deficiency. Then let me discuss the relevant medical literature – of which there is surprisingly little. Finally let me suggest why these cases of iron deficiency anemia are presenting now. While the focus will be on otherwise healthy men, analogous data on otherwise healthy women – who more commonly have been associated with iron deficiency – will be available for comparison in an endnote.

Please note in the following cases that lab data suggestive of a non-psychiatric diagnosis frequently was already on file but not acted upon. Please also note that something as simple as a "complete blood count" frequently provided sufficient information; that is, that while more "exotic" lab tests might be useful for confirmation of the diagnosis, frequently they were not really needed.

Brief Case Reports:

Male Patient #1: [censored]. Lab results on file 2 months earlier: [censored]. New lab results: [censored].

Male Patient #2: [censored]. New lab results: [censored].

Male Patient #3: [censored]. New lab results: [censored].

Male Patient #4: [censored]. Lab results available on file 5 months earlier:[censored].New lab results: [censored].

Male Patient #5: [censored]. New lab results: [censored].

Male Patient #6: [censored]. Lab results already on file 9 months earlier: [censored]. New lab results: [censored].

Male Patient #7: [censored]. New lab results:[censored].

Male Patient #8: [censored]. New lab results: [censored].

Male Patient #9: [censored]. New lab results: [censored].

Male Patient #10: [censored]. New lab results: [censored].

Discussion:

Of the 10 male patients cited, note that 50% self-diagnosed "depression," that 20% self-diagnosed "anxiety," and 60% spoke of sleep disorder. It would not have been surprising if at least 20% had self-diagnosed "attention-deficit disorder". Of the 10 patients cited, note that 30% had lab data already on file that suggested iron deficiency.

Medical articles focusing on iron deficiency in otherwise healthy young men are almost non-existent – especially in contrast to the plethora of such articles focusing on otherwise healthy young women. A study published in early 2009 found a 14.9% incidence of iron deficiency in 18 year old Israeli men; a similar study published in late 2005 found an 18% incidence; a small study published in early 2005 found a 6% incidence in athletic North American men; a smaller study published in early 2004 found a 15% incidence in athletic Israeli men. Even if only the lowest number – 6% – is taken into account, the conclusion is that iron deficiency in otherwise healthy young men is not as rare as might be assumed.

Regarding iron deficiency correlating with cognitive disabilities, a study published in early 2007 found that Egyptian young adults with low hemoglobin levels performed worse than a control group on the Mini-

Mental State Examination, the Wechsler memory scale revised, and the Wechsler Adult Intelligence Scale revised – but also showed improvement with treatment. Regarding iron deficiency correlating with emotional disabilities, a study published in late 2007 found that iron deficiency appears to be more prevalent in otherwise healthy young men who attempt suicide. While only about 6% – and probably a larger number – of young men have iron deficiency, the cognitive and emotional consequences are not insignificant. Clearly there is much more work to be done in this area.

So why are so many patients – especially young men – suddenly presenting with the erroneous psychiatric self-diagnosis of "anxiety" or "depression" when iron deficiency is more likely the primary problem? Let me present only two possibilities – fully understanding that there may be additional explanations (strenuous physical exercise, for example).

The number of westerners consuming large quantities of caffeine – in coffee, tea, and so-called "energy drinks" – grew exponentially after about 1995. While several fatigue combating potions most popular in an earlier era – such as "Irn Bru" and "Geritol" – specifically sought to counteract iron deficiency, those from the current era are more likely to cause it. A study published in early 1983 noted that iron absorption from a hamburger meal was reduced 39% by pairing it with a cup of coffee and 64% by pairing it with a cup of tea. Subsequent studies confirmed this finding and recommended ways to get around the problem, such as adding vitamin C or oily fish to the meal or confining the caffeinated drink to before rather than during or after the meal. The impact of caffeine on iron absorption is dose related, so that the more potent the beverage the likely it is to promote iron deficiency.

Similarly, the number of westerners using "proton pump inhibitors" to counteract "heart burn" grew exponentially after about 2005. Unfortunately, these gastric acid reducing medications also reduce the absorption of vitamins B-12, C, and D as well as iron and magnesium. While indigestion can be debilitating, causing vitamin and iron deficiency can be equally so. A study published in early 2009 summarized much of the data on this.

These comments – on high-dose caffeine and on proton pump inhibitors – only suggest rather than prove why so many patients are presenting with iron deficiency masquerading as "anxiety" or "depression". These comments underscore, however, the importance of asking about nutritional habits and non-psychotropic medications when evaluating self-diagnosed "psychiatric" patients – especially young males.

As a final note, it is worth remembering that iron deficiency – even without anemia – has real consequences on the economic part of patients' overall well-being. Data published in early 2001 (extrapolated from field data published in early 1994) suggested that iron deficiency correlated with the following decreases in productivity: 4% in primarily cognitive work, 5% in light manual labor, and 17% in heavy manual labor. Being less productive in the workplace might contribute realistically to a patient's self-diagnosis of "depression" or "anxiety" – even if, in the best of all worlds, the most optimal first presentation would not be to a psychiatrist's office.

> "an erroneous notion of causation, ... accepting any condition that may be singled out and changed by therapy as the genuine cause." Scott Buchanan

To reiterate, that a patient complains of "depression" or "anxiety" does not mean that "depression" or "anxiety" is the only – or even the primary – problem. Just as acute or chronic "anti-depressant deficiency" or "anxiolytic deficiency" may not be the whole story, iron deficiency may not be the whole story yet an important factor to take into consideration nonetheless.

References:
Yakovlev PI. in <u>Manual of Military Neuropsychiatry</u>, Solomon HC & Yakovlev PI, editors. Philadelphia: W.B. Saunders Co, 1944. p.65.

Wiechers I, Smith FA, Stern TA. "A Guide to the Judicious Use of Laboratory Tests and Diagnostic Procedures in Psychiatric Practice." Psychiatric Times. May 2010;27(5):48-51, p.50.

Brumfitt W. "Primary iron-deficiency anaemia in young men." Q J Med. 1960 Jan;29:1-18, p.1.

Mikawa Y, Mizobuchi S, Egi M, Morita K. "Low serum concentrations of vitamin b6 and iron are related to panic attack and hyperventilation attack." Acta Med Okayama. 2013 Apr;67(2):99-104; "…We measured each parameter in 21 PA [panic attack] or HVA [hyperventilation attack] patients and compared the values with those from 20 volunteers. We found that both Vit B6 and iron levels were significantly lower in the PA/HVA group than in the volunteer group. …"

Chen MH, Su TP, Chen YS, Hsu JW, Huang KL, Chang WH, Chen TJ, Bai YM. "Association between psychiatric disorders and iron deficiency anemia among children and adolescents: a nationwide population-based study." BMC Psychiatry. 2013 Jun 4;13:161; "… Adolescents with IDA [iron deficiency anemia] were significantly associated with unipolar depressive disorder …, BD [bipolar disorder] …, anxiety disorder …, ADHD [attention deficit hyperactivity disorder] … . [the overall study was of 2957 children & adolescents].

Yi S, Nanri A, Poudel-Tandukar K, Nonaka D, Matsushita Y, Hori A, Mizoue T. "Association between serum ferritin concentrations and depressive symptoms in Japanese municipal employees." Psychiatry Res. 2011 Oct 30;189(3):368-72; "…312 men and 216 women [ages not given] working in two municipal offices in Japan. Depressive symptoms were assessed by using the Center for Epidemiologic Studies Depression (CES-D) scale. In men, increased prevalence of depressive symptoms (defined by using a cutoff value of ≥ 19) was significantly associated with decreased levels of serum ferritin. … No significant association was detected in women. …"

Armed Forces Health Surveillance Center (AFHSC). "Iron deficiency anemia, active component, U.S. Armed Forces, 2002-2011." MSMR. 2012 Jul;19(7):17-21; [pregnancy-related anemia excluded; "traumatic injuries were infrequently associated"] "… the overall incidence rate was 7.1 per 10,000 person-years [male: 3.4; female: 29.5]. The annual incidence rates increased in both males and females during the period. ... Most (85.3%) incident cases had no additional encounters for IDA one year or more after their incident encounter. ..." [this was chart-review rather than systematic determination; these incidence rates must be viewed as minimums]

Yanovich R, Merkel D, Israeli E, Evans RK, Erlich T, Moran DS. "Anemia, iron deficiency, and stress fractures in female combatants during 16 months." J Strength Cond Res. 2011 Dec;25(12):3412-21; the male patients cited in the current manuscript were controls.

Merkel D, Huerta M, Grotto I, Blum D, Rachmilewitz E, Fibach E, Epstein Y, Shpilberg O. "Incidence of anemia and iron deficiency in strenuously trained adolescents: results of a longitudinal follow-up study. J Adolesc Health. 2009 Sep;45(3):286-91.

Merkel D, Huerta M, Grotto I, Blum D, Tal O, Rachmilewitz E, Fibach E, Epstein Y, Shpilberg O. "Prevalence of iron deficiency and anemia among strenuously trained adolescents. J Adolesc Health. 2005 Sep;37(3):220-3.

Sinclair LM, Hinton PS. "Prevalence of iron deficiency with and without anemia in recreationally active men and women. J Am Diet Assoc. 2005 Jun;105(6):975-8.

Dubnov G, Constantini NW. "Prevalence of iron depletion and anemia in top-level basketball players. Int J Sport Nutr Exerc Metab. 2004 Feb;14(1):30-7.

Li Y, Dai Q, Torres ME, Zhang J. "Gender-specific association between iron status and the history of attempted suicide: implications for gender paradox of suicidal behaviors." Prog Neuropsychopharmacol Biol Psychiatry. 2007 Oct 1;31(7):1429-35.

Soto-Insuga V, Calleja ML, Prados M, Castaño C, Losada R, Ruiz-Falcó ML. ["Role of iron in the treatment of attention deficit-hyperactivity disorder."][Article in Spanish] An Pediatr (Barc). An Pediatr (Barc). 2013 Oct;79(4):230-5; "...Those with ferritin ≤ 30ng/ml were treated with ferrous sulphate (4mg/kg/day) for 3 months ... . 60 patients, with a mean age of 9.02 years (range: 6-14), were analysed. The inattentive subtype was the most frequent one (53.3%). Almost two-thirds (63.3%) had iron deficiency, which was more frequent among the inattentive group (38 vs

22, P<.02). ... The probability of complete response after treatment with iron was higher in inattentive patients with ADHD (P=.02). ..."

Lahat E, Heyman E, Livne A, Goldman M, Berkovitch M, Zachor D. "Iron deficiency in children with attention deficit hyperactivity disorder." Isr Med Assoc J. 2011 Sep;13(9):530-3. "... Several studies have suggested that iron deficiency may be related to the pathophysiology of attention deficit hyperactivity disorder (ADHD) due to the role of iron in the production of dopamine and noradrenaline. ... The study group included 113 newly referred ADHD children aged 5-15 years (mean age 8.8 +/- 2.7).... Ferritin levels were below 20 ng/ml in 67 children (59%)

Calarge C, Farmer C, Disilvestro R, Arnold LE. "Serum ferritin and amphetamine response in youth with attention-deficit/hyperactivity disorder." J Child Adolesc Psychopharmacol. 2010 Dec;20(6):495-502; "... Fifty-two participants (83% males) had a mean age of 10 years ... . Serum ferritin was inversely correlated with baseline inattention, hyperactivity/ impulsivity, and total ADHD symptom scores. ..." [similar data are not yet available for adults]

Kahlon N, Gandhi A, Mondal S, Narayan S. "Effect of iron deficiency anemia on audiovisual reaction time in adolescent girls." Indian J Physiol Pharmacol. 2011 Jan-Mar;55(1):53-9; the subjects were 17-19 years old.

Morck TA, Lynch SR, Cook JD. "Inhibition of food iron absorption by coffee." Am J Clin Nutr. 1983 Mar;37(3):416-20.

Zijp IM, Korver O, Tijburg LB. "Effect of tea and other dietary factors on iron absorption." Crit Rev Food Sci Nutr.2000 Sep;40(5):371-98.

McColl KE. "Effect of proton pump inhibitors on vitamins and iron." Am J Gastroenterol. 2009 Mar;104 Suppl 2:S5-9.

Horton S, Levin C. "Commentary on 'Evidence that iron deficiency anemia causes reduced work capacity'." J Nutr. 2001 Feb;131(2S-2):691S-696S.

Tansarli GS, Karageorgopoulos DE, Kapaskelis A, Gkegkes I, Falagas ME. "Iron deficiency and susceptibility to infections: evaluation of the clinical evidence." Eur J Clin Microbiol Infect Dis. 2013 Oct;32(10):1253-8; "... Six studies (including a total of 1,422 participants) met the inclusion criteria ... The limited available evidence suggests that individuals with iron deficiency and those with iron deficiency anemia may be more susceptible to infections than patients with normal iron status. ...”

Buchanan S. The Doctrine of Signatures: A Defense of Theory in Medicine. 2nd edition [1938; 1st edition was 1935]. reprinted, Urbana: University of Illinois Press, 1991. p.71.

Endnote:

For comparison with the above-cited cases in men, please consider the following similar cases of iron deficiency in women:

Brief Case Reports:

Female Patient #1: [censored]. New lab results: [censored].

Female Patient #2: [censored]. Lab results already on file 3 months earlier: [censored]. New lab results: [censored].

Female Patient #3: [censored]. New lab results: [censored].

Female Patient #4: [censored]. Lab results on file 6 weeks earlier – which were attributed to [censored]. Lab results on file 3 weeks earlier - when fatigue was attributed to [censored]. New lab result: [censored]. This patient disappeared to immediate follow-up, but it was ascertained that 1 year later she was placed on an anxiolytic for [censored] – and still had not been placed on iron, even though the following lab results had been obtained 1 month before: [censored]. It is hard to grasp how so much available data could be ignored.

Female Patient #5: [censored]. New lab results: [censored].

Female Patient #6: [censored]. Lab results on file 15 months earlier: [censored]. Lab results on file 1 month earlier: [censored].

Female Patient #7: [censored]. Lab results already on file 18 months earlier: [censored]. New lab results: [censored].

Female Patient #8: [censored]. New lab results: [censored].

Female Patient #9: [censored]. Lab results already on file 1 year earlier: [censored]. New lab results: [censored].

Female Patient #10: [censored]. New lab results: [censored].

Discussion:

Of the 10 female patients cited, note that 80% self-diagnosed "depression," that 10% self-diagnosed "anxiety," and 20% spoke of sleep disorder. It would not have been surprising if at least 20% had self-diagnosed "attention-deficit disorder". Of the 10 patients cited, note that 50% had lab data already on file that suggested iron deficiency.

Reference:

Blanton CA, Green MW, Kretsch MJ. "Body iron is associated with cognitive executive planning function in college women." Br J Nutr. 2013 Mar 14;109(5):906-13; "… Healthy, non-anaemic undergraduate women (n 42) provided a blood sample and completed a standardised cognitive test battery … . Fe status in the absence of anaemia is positively associated with central executive function in otherwise healthy college women."

II. Pyridoxine (B-6) Deficiency.

"In humans, the [pyridoxine] deficiency syndrome is ill-defined. It is characterized by weakness, irritability and nervousness, insomnia, and difficulty in walking."
Carolyn D. Berdanier

"there is biochemical evidence of inadequate vitamin B6 nutritional status in 10-25 per cent of the population."
David A. Bender

A significant number of patients present with the erroneous psychiatric self-diagnosis of "depression" or "anxiety" when pyridoxine deficiency is more likely the primary problem. Recognizing this has been impeded by the continuing general assumption that pyridoxine deficiency is rare – although accumulating data suggest otherwise. Almost the entire literature on pyridoxine deficiency in humans has been published during the last fifty years. Also, while correcting pyridoxine deficiency may be worth the effort in terms of medical benefit to a self-defined suffering patient, until recently it was unlikely to have been worth the effort in terms of financial benefit to a pharmaceutical company. [In early 2009, however, the United States Food and Drug Administration recognized a company's patent on one version of B-6, "pyridoxamine dihydrochloride"; in early 2010 another company petitioned the US FDA to recognize its patent on another version of B-6, "pyridoxal 5-phosphate".]

First let me present several of the most illustrative cases seen in an outpatient psychiatric practice over the last three years; overall, about five per cent of the newly evaluated patients were found to have pyridoxine deficiency. Then let me discuss the relevant medical literature

– of which there is surprisingly little. Finally let me suggest why these cases of pyridoxine deficiency are presenting now.

Please note in the following cases that lab data suggestive of a non-psychiatric diagnosis frequently was already on file but not acted upon. Please also note that something as simple as a "complete blood count" in conjunction with a "comprehensive metabolic profile" frequently provided sufficient information; that is, that while more a "exotic" lab test – a pyridoxine level – would be needed for confirmation of the diagnosis, frequently one could deduce it – by the rarity of folate deficiency and the presence of a known normal cobalamin (B-12) or methylmalonic acid (MMA) level in the presence of both macrocytosis and a low aspartate aminotransferase (AST) level [previously known as a serum glutamic-oxaloacetic transaminase (SGOT) level]. [The presence of a definitely low AST did not always correctly predict pyridoxine deficiency, and the literature suggests that a definitely low alanine aminotransferase (ALT) level would be a more sensitive indicator if and when it is seen.] This clinical approach makes intuitive sense to those who work in medical chemistry laboratories as the functional assay for pyridoxine is based on measuring the level of erythrocyte AST [or ALT] activity both before and after stimulation of the blood sample with pyridoxal phosphate [PLP].

Please also note that in the following cases a low pyridoxine level appears to correlate with macrocytosis rather than with microcytosis. Most of the medical literature – most of it quite old and using non-human subjects – suggests that the opposite would be the case – that microcytosis would be expected. Just as one can have "iron deficiency without anemia," analogously one can have "pyridoxine deficiency without anemia" – at least in humans – despite the fact that red cell parameters can hint that pyridoxine deficiency might be present. In a classic experiment published in 1950, only one of eight human subjects in whom pyridoxine deficiency was induced developed anemia, and on closer scrutiny the anemia in that one subject appeared to be secondary to folate deficiency. Since pyridoxine deficiency sometimes does correlate with reduced iron absorption, it could be that the somewhat sparse older literature was describing cases in which gross malnutrition had produced a combination of deficiencies; this question needs to be resolved by studies on humans who definitely are not iron deficient.

With the following cases, frequently the "complete blood count" and "comprehensive metabolic profile" results had come back while the patient was still in the clinic building – so that it was not that difficult to have the patient called back to the lab for a pyridoxine level. [During the time span of this study, with this population, cobalamin deficiency was not that uncommon, but pyridoxine deficiency was confirmed thirty times more frequently than was folate deficiency.]

Let me add a few more words about diagnosing pyridoxine deficiency from very basic laboratory tests. There are very few medical conditions [eg, azotemia, chronic renal dialysis, pregnancy, hypogonadism] that might cause an isolated low AST value and fewer still [eg, urinary tract infection, malnutrition] that might cause an isolated low ALT value; in fact, in either case a high value generally is more cause for concern, and a lowered value generally generates comment only because it once was higher. A study published in 2007 found that even raised ALT values were ignored if the elevation were only mild or intermittent, despite the very real clinical consequences. When an isolated definitely low AST [or ALT] value is spotted, however, a physician might want to scan to see if there is an accompanying high mean corpuscular hemoglobin [MCH] level – which would suggest that pyridoxine deficiency might be present. Most physicians, one must suspect, would think of AST [and ALT] in the context of organ pathology rather than in the context of vitamin deficiency.

Brief Case Reports:
Female Patient #1: [censored]. Lab results already on file from 3 weeks earlier: [censored]. That is, the high homocysteine level was only possibly due to vitamin B-12 deficiency and was definitely not due to folate deficiency – which raised the question of whether it could be due to pyridoxine deficiency. New lab results: [censored].

Female Patient #2: [censored]. New lab results: [censored].

Female Patient #3: [censored]. Lab results already on file 6 months earlier: [censored]. New lab results: [censored]. That is, the high homocysteine level was definitely not due to either vitamin B-12 deficiency or folate deficiency but was due to pyridoxine deficiency.

Female Patient #4: [censored]. Lab results already on file 1 month before: [censored]. Lab result on file from 5 months before: [censored]. New lab results: [censored].

Female Patient #5: [censored]. Lab result on file 6 months before: [censored]. Lab results from 6 weeks before: [censored]. New lab results: [censored].

Female Patient #6: [censored]. Lab results already on file 1 year before: [censored]. New lab results: [censored].

Female Patient #7: [censored]. Lab results on file 5 months earlier: [censored]. New lab result: [censored].

Female Patient #8: [censored]. New lab results: [censored].

Female Patient #9: [censored]. Lab results already on file 2 weeks before: [censored]. New lab results: [censored].

Female Patient # 10: [censored]. Lab results already on file 6 months before: [censored]. New lab results: [censored].

Male Patient #1: [censored]. New lab results: [censored].

Male Patient #2: [censored]. New lab results: [censored].

Male Patient #3: [censored]. New lab results: [censored].

Male Patient #4: [censored]. New lab results: [censored].

Male Patient #5: [censored]. Lab results already on file 6 months earlier: [censored]. New lab results: [censored].

Male Patient #6: [censored]. New lab results: [censored].

Discussion:

Of the 6 male patients with pyridoxine deficiency cited in this convenience sample, note that 50% self-diagnosed "depression" and that 50% self-diagnosed a mixed "depression/ anxiety". Of the 10 female patients cited, note that 50% self-diagnosed "depression," that 30% self-diagnosed a mixed "depression/ anxiety, and that 20% self-diagnosed "anxiety". That is, while the numbers are small, the suggestion is that female patients might be more likely than male patients to experience pyridoxine deficiency as including anxiety. Of the 16 patients cited, note that 7 had lab data already on file that suggested pyridoxine deficiency.

Medical articles focusing on pyridoxine deficiency in otherwise healthy patients are rare. A study published in early 2008 found an 11% prevalence of pyridoxine deficiency in North Americans who used supplements and a 24% prevalence in those who did not. Women of childbearing age were significantly more deficient – especially those who were using or had used oral contraceptives. When one adds that pyridoxine is a cofactor for 5-hydroxytryptophan decarboxylase and aromatic-L-amino-acid decarboxylase, two enzymes involved in the biosynthesis of serotonin, a chemical considered important for mood stabilization, then the 11% and greater prevalence of pyridoxine deficiency becomes potentially even more important. A study published in early 2008 found that North Americans taking a pyridoxine supplement for 6 months were 63% more likely to have a reduction in Beck Depression Inventory scores than those who did not. Another study published in early 2010, of 3,503 older North Americans, found that for every additional 10mg of pyridoxine consumed over an average of 7 years there was a 2% drop in the incidence of depression per year. Clearly there is much more work to be done in this area.

So why are so many patients – especially young males [that is, patients not using birth control pills] – suddenly presenting with the erroneous psychiatric self-diagnosis of "anxiety" or "depression" when pyridoxine deficiency is more likely the primary problem? Let me discuss several possibilities. Some of the sparse literature suggests the role of excessive intake of either alcohol or caffeine, but this factor was present in only 4 of the above-cited 15 cases; in fact, if anything, the other 11 cases were notable for their avoidance of both alcohol and caffeine.

Pyridoxine deficiency also has been cited as correlating with zinc deficiency, as the enzyme required for the phosphorylation reactions between the various forms of pyridoxine requires zinc for activation.

While a number of somewhat low zinc levels were seen in this patient population during the time of this study, cases of definite pyridoxine deficiency were 5 times more common.

High protein intake can lead to pyridoxine deficiency, and that might have been a factor in about half the cases in this generally athletic population. While it is doubtful that high protein intake accounts primarily for the notably increased incidence of pyridoxine deficiency, it must be considered when encountered in the context of high intake of alcohol, caffeine, or both.

One possibility that definitely might bear further consideration is the ubiquity of both frozen food and overcooked food – including food that is frozen for an extensive period of time before being simmered for an extensive period of time – as might occur in certain cafeteria or other self-serve settings. For the specific population discussed in this survey, the destruction of pyridoxine – a fragile vitamin – by long-term freezing then by long-term heating much be considered the most likely cause of a sudden increase in definite cases of deficiency.

To reiterate, that a patient complains of "depression" or "anxiety" does not mean that "depression" or "anxiety" is the only – or even the primary – problem. Just as acute or chronic "anti-depressant deficiency" or "anxiolytic deficiency" may not be the whole story, pyridoxine deficiency may not be the whole story yet an important factor to take into consideration nonetheless. While some of these patients would have chosen to consult with a mental health professional even if their pyridoxine deficiency already had been adequately treated, it is doubtful that all would have chosen that route.

References:

Berdanier CD. "Pyridoxine, pyridoxamine, pyridoxic acid." in CRC Desk Reference for Nutrition, 2nd ed. NY: CRC/ Taylor & Francis, 2006. pp.369-375, p.374.

Bender DA. "Vitamin B6 requirements and recommendations." Eur J

Clin Nutr. 1989 May;43(5):289-309, p.289.

McPherson RA & Pincus MR, editors. Henry's Clinical Diagnosis and Management by Laboratory Methods, 21st ed. NY: Elsevier/ Saunders, 2003, p.381.

Raica N Jr, Sauberlich HE. "Blood cell transaminase activity in human B6 deficiency." Amer J Clin Nutr. 1964 Aug;15:67-72.

Rej R, Fasce CF Jr, Vanderlinde RE. "Increased aspartate aminotransferase activity of serum after in vitro supplementation with pyridoxal phosphate." Clin Chem. 1973 Jan;19(1):92-8.

Nanji AA. "Decreased activity of commonly measured serum enzymes: causes and clinical significance." Am J Med Technol. 1983 Apr;49(4):241-5.

Mueller JF, Vilter RW. "Pyridoxine deficiency in human beings induced by desoxypyridoxine." J Clin Invest. 1950 Feb;29(2):193-201.

Pocha C, Gaylord K, Maliakal B, Rodgers JB. "Evaluating primary care providers' responses to serum alanine aminotransferase elevations." Federal Practitioner. 2007;24(7):44-57,71; only 6 of the 449 cases reviewed – 1% – received "an acceptable workup" of "mild and intermittent" elevation all the way to diagnosis.

Morris MS, Picciano MF, Jacques PF, Selhub J. "Plasma pyridoxal 5'-phosphate in the US population: the National Health and Nutrition Examination Survey, 2003-2004." Am J Clin Nutr. 2008 May;87(5):1446-54.

Allen GF, Neergheen V, Oppenheim M, Fitzgerald JC, Footitt E, Hyland K, Clayton PT, Land JM, Heales SJ. "Pyridoxal 5'-phosphate deficiency causes a loss of aromatic L-amino acid decarboxylase in patients and human neuroblastoma cells, implications for aromatic L-amino acid decarboxylase and vitamin B(6) deficiency states." J Neurochem. 2010 Jul;114(1):87-96.

Mikawa Y, Mizobuchi S, Egi M, Morita K. "Low serum concentrations of vitamin b6 and iron are related to panic attack and hyperventilation attack." Acta Med Okayama. 2013 Apr;67(2):99-104; "…We measured each parameter in 21 PA [panic attack] or HVA [hyperventilation attack] patients and compared the values with those from 20 volunteers. We found that both Vit B6 and iron levels were significantly lower in the PA/HVA group than in the volunteer group. ..."

Merrill RM, Taylor P, Aldana SG. "Coronary Health Improvement Project (CHIP) is associated with improved nutrient intake and decreased depression." Nutrition. 2008 Apr;24(4):314-21.

Skarupski KA, Tangney C, Li H, Ouyang B, Evans DA, Morris MC. "Longitudinal association of vitamin B-6, folate, and vitamin B-12 with depressive symptoms among older adults over time." Am J Clin Nutr. 2010 Jun 2.

III. Zinc Deficiency

"… intense metabolic and mental demands, as well as exposure to various immune challenges. Some of these factors may affect … dietary zinc requirements."
James P. McClung

"… less obvious, but more insidious in outcomes, are longer-term changes that can result from poor zinc status, such as … irritability, anxiety, depression, difficulty with concentration and cognitive function, impaired learning, or other psychoneurological conditions."
Mitchell Bebel Stargrove, Jonathan Treasure &
Dwight L. McKee

A significant number of patients present with the erroneous psychiatric self-diagnosis of "depression" or "anxiety" when zinc deficiency is more likely the primary problem. Recognizing this has been impeded by the infrequency with which serum or plasma [more accurate] zinc levels are obtained, although a growing literature on the role of zinc in neurologic, immunologic, endocrinologic, orthopedic, dermatologic, and gastrointestinal conditions may begin changing this. Almost the entire literature on zinc deficiency in humans has been published during the last fifty years. Appreciating the frequency of zinc deficiency has been impeded further by an awareness that contamination carried on other mineral supplements can produce a spuriously high zinc level, while the reverse situation is more to the point – that only hypoalbuminemia – most likely to be encountered in an obviously ill patient – is known to produce a spuriously low zinc level. That is, while a high zinc level might be suspect, a low zinc level is not to be ignored. Also, while correcting zinc deficiency may be worth the effort in terms of medical benefit to a self-defined suffering patient, it is unlikely to be worth the effort in terms of financial benefit to a pharmaceutical company.

First let me present several of the most illustrative cases seen in an outpatient psychiatric practice over the last three years; overall, a little over one per cent of the newly evaluated patients were found to have zinc deficiency – with the level generally being ordered in the face of some known supposedly non-psychiatric condition. Then let me discuss the relevant medical literature – of which there is surprisingly little. Finally let me suggest some possible reasons why these cases of zinc deficiency are presenting now.

Please note in the following cases that clinical data suggestive of a non-psychiatric diagnosis frequently was available in the opening "psychiatric chief complaint," the history of medical illness, or both – but that the operant word here is "suggestive" – as there is no known definitive characteristic associated with zinc deficiency.

It must be emphasized that in each of the cases being cited it was a non-psychiatric piece of data that led to the obtaining of a zinc level. Furthermore, it must be noted that 5 out of 11 – that is, 45% – of the following out-patients had at least one other definite deficiency – and that 2 others of the cohort were trending toward additional deficiency – with hypomagnesemia most commonly being the extra factor. For 3 of the cases one is hard-pressed to conclude which is the primary deficiency. Thus these 11 case histories are more medically complex than one might expect – yet all received the bulk of their care – including encouragement toward further non-psychiatric evaluation – via the mental health clinic. It was only in retrospect that a common psychiatric theme – to be discussed later – was noted among the cases assembled.

Brief Case Reports:
Male Patient #1: [censored]. The zinc level was ordered because he had variable effectiveness from his use of amphetamine prescribed to reduce difficulty staying on task as well as to reduce irritability/

impulsivity. New lab results: [censored].

Male Patient #2: [censored]. The zinc level was ordered because he had had "notable hair loss for 2 years." New lab results: [censored].

Male Patient #3: [censored]. The zinc level was ordered because there was a question of chronic low-grade anorexia. Lab results on file 14 months earlier: [censored].

Female Patient #1: [censored]. The zinc level was ordered because of her "problems with inattentiveness." New lab results: [censored].

Female Patient #2: [censored]. The zinc level was ordered because of her attention problems, alopecia, and beginning hypothyroidism. New lab results: [censored]. Lab results 6 weeks later noting hypocalcemia: [censored]. Is this *primarily* hypocalcemia or nascent hypothyroidism or zinc deficiency or none of the above?

Female Patient #3: [censored]. The zinc level was ordered because of her significant alopecia. New lab results: [censored].

Female Patient #4: [censored]. The zinc level was ordered because she had had "notable hair loss since age 15". Is this *primarily* hypomagnesemia or hyponatremia or hypocalcemia or spurious zinc deficiency [because of the hypoalbuminemia] – or none of the above?

Male Patient #4: [censored]. The zinc level was ordered because of his dermatologic issue. New lab results: [censored].

Female Patient #5: [censored]. The zinc level was ordered because of her vague neurologic symptoms and significant anorexia. Lab results already on file 4.5 months earlier: [censored]. Intriguingly, apparently she had not been placed on any vitamins or minerals. New lab results 3 days before the psychiatric evaluation [censored]. Is this *primarily* hypomagnesaemia or hyponatremia or hyperglobulinemia or iron deficiency or zinc deficiency – or none of the above? The patient worked in psychotherapy the entire time but moved away at the end of 1 more month, taking a copy of her lab results with her. The medical clinic continued to insist that her symptoms were "non-organic and probably benign".

Female Patient #6: [censored]. The zinc level was ordered because of her significant hyperactivity. New lab results: [censored].

Female Patient #7: [censored]. The zinc level was ordered because of her history of significant alopecia. New lab results; [censored].

Discussion:

Of the 11 patients with zinc deficiency cited in this convenience sample, note that about half self-diagnosed "depression" or something similar and that about half self-diagnosed "anxiety" or something similar. There was, however, an unusual quality to these self-assessments, with neither "depression" nor "anxiety" seeming quite adequate to describing the situations experienced.

Notice some of the words being used in these brief case histories: "like everything is out of my control" – "like no one was watching over me – like a protector" – "feeling overwhelmed" – "minimal effective and persistent control over his life" – "no one is looking out for my best interests" – "dependence/ independence conflicts" – "very sensitive to criticism and rejection" – "distancing in regard to fear" – "overwhelmed and demoralized" – "I'll be having thoughts about home – and I'll burst into tears" – "concerned about being overwhelmed by fear" – "began getting worried about everything" – "competent but notably insecure". The cases were collected without any psychological preconceptions whatsoever, so it came as quite a surprise to note that themes about vulnerability and not being taken care of were front and center.

None of these patients were viewed by themselves or others as severely or even moderately depressed or anxious in any classical sense. They were viewed as somehow "odd" – but not clearly as depressed or anxious in a manner with which others might easily identify; if fact, all seemed somewhat socially alienated.

Medical articles focusing on zinc deficiency in otherwise healthy patients are rare. A search of the medical literature did reveal that there is new interest in the role of zinc in the brain's processing of fear, plus that zinc levels correlate inversely with depression and attentiveness. No one else seems to have noted, however, the clustering of psychological concerns outlined here – vulnerability and not being taken care of – a clustering that is very different from other varieties of apparent depression mixed with anxiety. It must be observed, however, that many of the medical issues sometimes accompanying zinc deficiency – for example, inattentiveness, frequent sickness, hair loss, sexual decrement, bone brittleness, acne, and anorexia – do not exactly support a sense of security and self-esteem supporting independence. The conclusion is, however, if the patient has a definite neurologic, immunologic, endocrinologic, orthopedic, dermatologic, or gastrointestinal condition plus has clear concerns about vulnerability and not being taken care of, then one might want to consider ordering a zinc level.

Zinc deficiency is common in many of the so-called "Third World" countries – including Iraq and Afghanistan – but does occur in the United States – primarily because of some crop soils that have been over-fertilized with phosphates, which bind with zinc, or because of some patients' unbalanced over-consumption of cereal, legume, and nut proteins. Otherwise, it is not clear why this number of patients with zinc deficiency were encountered – especially since such a large number of them had multiple nutritional deficiencies. The entire situation clearly is not well-understood either here or abroad, but the World Health Organization and other governmental organizations have decided to move ahead with the use of zinc supplementation of select populations because of the empirically noted impact on reducing disease.

As a final note, it is worth remembering that zinc deficiency – even mild zinc deficiency – may have real consequences on patients' overall well-being. Data published in 2006-2007 noted that zinc supplementation could prevent exercise-induced reductions of both testosterone and thyroid hormones. Data published in late 2009 (following up on numerous animal studies) suggested that even mild zinc deficiency in otherwise healthy men correlated with increased DNA strand breaks in peripheral blood cells – changes that were ameliorated by adding dietary zinc.

To reiterate, that a patient complains of "depression" or "anxiety" does not mean that "depression" or "anxiety" is the only – or even the primary – problem. Just as acute or chronic "anti-depressant deficiency" or "anxiolytic deficiency" may not be the whole story, zinc deficiency may not be the whole story yet an important factor to take into consideration nonetheless. While some of these patients would have chosen to consult with a mental health professional even if their zinc deficiency already had been adequately treated, it is doubtful that all would have chosen that route.

References:
Mitchell W, Feldman F. "Neuropsychiatric aspects of hypokalemia." CMAJ. 1968 Jan 06;98:49-51; p.51.

McClung JP, Scrimgeour AG. "Zinc: an essential trace element with potential benefit to soldiers." Mil Med.2005 Dec;170(120(12):1048-52, p.1048.

Stargrove MB, Treasure J, and McKee DL. Herb, <u>Nutrient, and Drug Interactions: Clinical Implications and Therapeutic Strategies</u>. Elsevier/ Mosby, 2008. p.622.

Hambidge M. "Human zinc deficiency." J Nutr.2000 May;130(5S Suppl):1344S-9S; an overview of & introduction to "Zinc and Health: Current Status and Future Directions," a workshop convened in November 1998 by the [U.S.] National Institutes of Health.

Kodirov SA, Takizawa S, Joseph J, Kandel ER, Shumyatsky GP, Bolshakov VY. "Synaptically released zinc gates long-term potentiation in fear conditioning pathways." Proc Natl Acad Sci USA.2006 Oct 10;103(41):15218-23.

Ranjbar E, Kasaei MS, Mohammad-Shirazi M, Nasrollahzadeh J, Rashidkhani B, Shams J, Mostafavi SA, Mohammadi MR. "Effects of zinc supplementation in patients with major depression: a randomized clinical trial." Iran J Psychiatry. 2013 Jun;8(2):73-9; "…double-blind randomized clinical trial. Forty four patients with major depression were randomly assigned to groups receiving zinc supplementation and placebo. Patients in Zinc group received daily supplementation with 25 mg zinc adjunct to antidepressant; Selective Serotonin Reuptake Inhibitors (SSRIs), while the patients in placebo group received placebo with antidepressants (SSRIs) for twelve weeks. ... The mean score of Beck Depression Inventory reduced significantly compared to the placebo group at the end of 12th week ... ."

Swardfager W1, Herrmann N, Mazereeuw G, Goldberger K, Harimoto T, Lanctôt KL. "Zinc in depression: a meta-analysis." Biol Psychiatry. 2013 Dec 15;74(12):872-8. "... Seventeen studies, measuring peripheral blood zinc concentrations in 1643 depressed and 804 control subjects, were included. Zinc concentrations were approximately -1.85 µmol/L lower in depressed subjects ... . greater depression severity was associated with greater relative zinc deficiency ... ."

Swardfager W, Herrmann N, McIntyre RS, Mazereeuw G, Goldberger K, Cha DS, Schwartz Y, Lanctôt KL. "Potential roles of zinc in the pathophysiology and treatment of major depressive disorder." Neurosci Biobehav Rev. 2013 Jun;37(5):911-29; "... Neuronal zinc is concentrated exclusively within glutamatergic neurons, acting as an allosteric modulator of the N-methyl D-aspartate and other receptors that regulate excitatory neurotransmission and neuroplasticity. Zinc-containing neurons form extensive associational circuitry throughout the cortex, amygdala and hippocampus, which subserve mood regulation and cognitive functions. ... Clinically, serum zinc is lower in MDD [Major Depressive Disorder] .... Initial randomized trials suggest a benefit of zinc supplementation. ..."

McLoughlin IJ, Hodge JS. "Zinc in depressive disorder." Acta Psychiatr Scand.1990 Dec;82(6):451-3.

Maes M, D'Haese PC, Scharpé S, D'Hondt P, Cosyns P, De Broe ME. "Hypozincemia in depression." J Affect Disord. 1994 Jun;31(2):135-40 [Maes is a major investigator of the immune deficiency view of depression].

Siwek M, Dudek D, Paul IA, Sowa-Kucma M, Zieba A, Popik P, Pilc A, Nowak G. "Zinc supplementation augments efficacy of imipramine in treatment resistant patients: a double blind, placebo-controlled study." J Affect Disord. 2009 Nov;118(1-3):187-95.

Szewczyk B, Kubera M, Nowak G. "The role of zinc in neurodegenerative inflammatory pathways in depression." Prog Neuropsychopharmacol Biol Psychiatry. 2011 Apr 29;35(3):693-701

Siwek M, Dudek D, Schlegel-Zawadzka M, Morawska A, Piekoszewski W, Opoka W, Zięba A, Pilc A, Popik P, Nowak G. "Serum zinc level in depressed patients during zinc supplementation of imipramine treatment." J Affect Disord. 2010 Nov;126(3):447-52.; a placebo-controlled double-blind study; "… the serum zinc level was significantly lower (by 22%) in depressed patients than in healthy volunteers … . treatment-resistant patients demonstrated lower concentrations of zinc (by 14%) than treatment-non-resistant patients … . Serum zinc is a state marker of depression."

Yary T, Aazami S. "Dietary intake of zinc was inversely associated with depression." Biol Trace Elem Res. 2012 Mar;145(3):286-90; "…402 participants with a mean age of 32.54 ± 6.22 years, including 173 (43%) women and 229 (57%) men. …"

Sawada T, Yokoi K. "Effect of zinc supplementation on mood states in young women: a pilot study." Eur J Clin Nutr. 2010 Mar;64(3):331-3; "…a double-blind, randomized and placebo-controlled procedure. … Thirty women were placed randomly and in equal numbers into two groups, and they ingested one capsule containing multivitamins (MVs) or MV and 7 mg Zn daily for 10 weeks. Women who took MV and Zn showed a significant reduction in anger-hostility score … and depression-dejection score … in the Profile of Moods State (POMS) …, whereas women who took only MV did not. …"

Cope EC, Levenson CW. "Role of zinc in the development and treatment of mood disorders." Curr Opin Clin Nutr Metab Care. 2010 Nov;13(6):685-9.

Islam MR, Ahmed MU, Mitu SA, Islam MS, Rahman GK, Qusar MM, Hasnat A. "Comparative analysis of serum zinc, copper, manganese, iron, calcium, and magnesium level and complexity of interelement relations in generalized anxiety disorder patients." Biol Trace Elem Res. 2013 Jul;154(1):21-7; "…50 generalized anxiety disorder patients and 51 healthy volunteers. Patients were selected and recruited in the study with the help of a clinical psychologist by random sampling. … Significantly decreased … serum Zn concentration was found in the patient group compared to the control group … ."

Song CH, Kim YH, Jung KI. "Associations of zinc and copper levels in serum and hair with sleep duration in adult women." Biol Trace Elem Res. 2012 Oct;149(1):16-21; "...126 adult women were recruited in this cross-sectional study. Zn and Cu levels in the serum and hair were measured for each subject. ... The largest percentage of participants with optimal sleep duration was observed in the highest tertile of Zn/Cu ratio in the serum and hair ... ."

Russo AJ. "Decreased zinc and increased copper in individuals with anxiety." Nutr Metab Insights. 2011 Feb 7;4:1-5; "...Serum from 38 individuals with anxiety and 16 neurotypical age, gender and size similar controls were tested for plasma zinc and copper concentration using inductively-coupled plasma-mass spectrometry. ... These results suggest an association between [decreased] Zn plasma levels and individuals with anxiety, demonstrate that zinc therapy is effective in increasing zinc plasma levels, and show that zinc supplementation may play a role in improved symptoms."

Nahar Z, Azad MA, Rahman MA, Rahman MA, Bari W, Islam SN, Islam MS, Hasnat A. "Comparative analysis of serum manganese, zinc, calcium, copper and magnesium level in panic disorder patients." Biol Trace Elem Res. 2010 Mar;133(3):284-90; "...54 panic disorder patients and 52 healthy volunteers. Patients were recruited ... by random sampling. ... The serum concentration of Zn decreased significantly ... in patient group. ..."

Lepping P, Huber M. "Role of zinc in the pathogenesis of attention-deficit hyperactivity disorder: implications for research and treatment." CNS Drugs. 2010 Sep 1;24(9):721-8

Arnold LE, Bozzolo H, Holloway J, Cook A, DiSilvestro RA, Bozzolo DR, Crowl L, Ramadan Y, Williams C. "Serum zinc correlates with parent- and teacher-rated inattention in children with attention-deficit/hyperactivity disorder." J Child Adolesc Psychopharmacol.2005 Aug;15(4):628-36.

Arnold LE, Disilvestro RA, Bozzolo D, Bozzolo H, Crowl L, Fernandez S, Ramadan Y, Thompson S, Mo X, Abdel-Rasoul M, Joseph E. "Zinc for attention-deficit/hyperactivity disorder: placebo-controlled double-blind pilot trial alone and combined with amphetamine." J Child Adolesc Psychopharmacol. 2011 Feb;21(1):1-19; "... 52 children aged 6-

14 with DSM-IV ADHD … . Optimal mg/kg AMPH [amphetamine] dose with b.i.d. [15mg] zinc [gluconate] was 37% lower than with placebo. …"

Hubbs-Tait L, Kennedy TS, Droke EA, Belanger DM, Parker JR. "Zinc, iron, and lead: relations to head start children's cognitive scores and teachers' ratings of behavior." J Am Diet Assoc.2007 Jan;107(1):128-33.

Briefel RR, Bialostosky K, Kennedy-Stephenson J, McDowell MA, Ervin RB, Wright JD. "Zinc intake of the U.S. population: findings from the third National Health and Nutrition Examination Survey [NHANES], 1988-1994." J Nutr.2000 May;130(5S Suppl):1367S-73S.

Prasad AS. "Impact of the discovery of human zinc deficiency on health." J Am Coll Nutr. 2009 Jun;28(3):257-65.

Foster M, Samman S. "Zinc and regulation of inflammatory cytokines: implications for cardiometabolic disease." Nutrients. 2012 Jul;4(7):676-94; "… an increased demand for zinc in inflammatory conditions. The acute phase response includes a rapid decline in the plasma zinc concentration as a result of the redistribution of zinc into cellular compartments. Zinc deficiency influences the generation of cytokines, including IL [interleukin]-1β, IL-2, IL-6, and TNF [tumor necrosis factor]-α, and in response to zinc supplementation plasma cytokines exhibit a dose-dependent response. The mechanism of action may reflect the ability of zinc to either induce or inhibit the activation of NF-κB [nuclear factor-kappa B, a protein complex that controls the transcription of DNA]. …"

Hess SY, Lonnerdal B, Hotz C, Rivera JA, Brown KH. "Recent advances in knowledge of zinc nutrition and human health." Food Nutr Bull.2009 Mar;30(1 Suppl):S5-11.

Kilic M, Baltaci AK, Gunay M, Gökbel H, Okudan N, Cicioglu I. "The effect of exhaustion exercise on thyroid hormones and testosterone levels of elite athletes receiving oral zinc." Neuro Endocrinol Lett. 2006 Feb-Apr;27(1-2):247-52; "… 10 male wrestlers, who had been licensed wrestlers for at least 6 years. Mean age of the wrestlers who volunteered in the study was 18.70 +/- 2.4 years. All subjects were supplemented with oral zinc sulfate (3 mg/kg/day) for 4 weeks in addition to their normal diet. … exhaustion exercise led to a significant inhibition of both thyroid hormones and testosterone concentrations, but that 4-week zinc supplementation prevented this inhibition in wrestlers. In conclusion, physiological doses of zinc administration may benefit performance."

Kilic M. "Effect of fatiguing bicycle exercise on thyroid hormone and testosterone levels in sedentary males supplemented with oral zinc." Neuro Endocrinol Lett. 2007 Oct;28(5):681-5; "…10 volunteers (mean age, 19.47+/-1.7 years) who did not exercise. All subjects received supplements of oral zinc sulfate (3 mg/kg/day) for 4 weeks and their normal diets. … exercise decreases thyroid hormones and testosterone in sedentary men; however, zinc supplementation prevents this decrease. Administration of a physiologic dose of zinc can be beneficial to performance."

Song Y, Chung CS, Bruno RS, Traber MG, Brown KH, King JC, Ho E. "Dietary zinc restriction and repletion affects DNA integrity in healthy men." Am J Clin Nutr. 2009 Aug;90(2):321-8.

National Academy of Sciences (U.S.) (the Committee on Mineral Requirements for Cognitive and Physical Performance of Military Personnel, the Committee on Military Nutrition Research, and the Food and Nutrition Board). Mineral Requirements for Military Personnel: Levels Needed for Cognitive and Physical Performance during Garrison Training. Washington, D.C.: National Academies Press, 2006. [This is an excellent review of what is known – and not known – about the roles of calcium, copper, iron, magnesium, selenium, and zinc in human nutrition.]

IV. Severe Vitamin D Deficiency

"Vitamin D as a neuroactive compound, a prohormone, is highly active ... in a variety of structures, including the brain. Vitamin D insufficiency is not rare. ... The central nervous system is increasingly recognized as a target organ for vitamin D via its wide-ranging hormonal effects, including the induction of proteins such as nerve growth factor."
Steven J. Kiraly, Michael A. Kiraly, Rick D. Hawe, Naila Makhani

"there is ample biological evidence to suggest an important role for vitamin D in brain development and function. However, direct effects of vitamin D inadequacy on cognition/behavior in human or rodent systems appear to be subtle ... ."
Joyce C. McCann, Bruce N. Ames

An amazing number of patients present with the erroneous psychiatric self-diagnosis of "depression" or "anxiety" when _severe_ vitamin D deficiency – a "total 25-hydroxy vitamin D level" ["calcidiol" – the only recommended test] in the range of 5 to 13, where the "normal" range is defined (at minimum) – as above 20 NG/ML – is more likely the primary problem. Recognizing this has been impeded by the odd circumstance that severe vitamin D deficiency is more likely to correlate with a mild, vague, somewhat bland variety of depression rather than with a severe, definite, somewhat dramatic variety of depression. While such patients use the word "depression" and sometimes add the word "anxiety" or the word "tension" to try to describe how they are feeling, one gets the sense that they are not sure that their situations merit consulting with a psychiatrist; they just know that something is not right. That is, these are patients who would be rejected by most clinical research projects trying to prove that this or that pharmaceutical intervention is effective. To make matters worse, it may take months – or even years – to correct severe vitamin D deficiency – that is, to move a patient's correlating emotional condition from "mild depression" to "non-depression".

While correcting severe vitamin D deficiency may be worth the effort in terms of medical benefit to a self-defined suffering patient, it is unlikely to be worth the effort in terms of financial benefit to a pharmaceutical company. An interesting confirmation of this is an article published in late 2009 while lamented that while supplemental vitamin D might improve mild depression there was no evidence thus far that it could improve moderate-to-severe depression. In other words, the attitude essentially was "why bother?" – fully discounting that the somatic consequences of significant vitamin D deficiency might impair daily functioning and thus mood.

First let me present several of the most illustrative cases seen in an outpatient psychiatric practice over the last three years; overall, about twelve per cent of the newly evaluated patients were found to have vitamin D deficiency and about six per cent were found to have severe vitamin D deficiency. Then let me discuss the relevant medical literature – of which there is surprisingly little. Finally let me suggest some possible reasons why these cases of severe vitamin D deficiency are presenting now. While the focus will be on the most severe cases of vitamin D deficiency, analogous data will be presented in an endnote on an equal number of only slightly less severe cases – none of which had a level of higher than 19 NG/ML.

Please note in the following cases that clinical data suggestive of a non-psychiatric diagnosis frequently was available in the opening "psychiatric chief complaint," the history of medical illness, or both – but that the operant word here is "suggestive" – as there is no known definitive characteristic associated with severe vitamin D deficiency. It must be emphasized that in each of the cases being cited it was a non-psychiatric piece of data that led to the obtaining of a 25-hydroxy vitamin D level. It was only in retrospect that a common psychiatric theme – to be discussed later – was noted among the cases assembled.

Let me emphasize that only the most severe cases have been chosen for consideration in this study. Psychiatric skepticism regarding even a correlation – let alone any implication of causation – between vitamin D deficiency and depression appears to be so high that focusing on anything less than the most severe cases would be a waste of effort. While patients having a 25-hydroxy vitamin D level of at least 20 NG/ML currently are defined as "normal," most experts in the field would argue that any level less than 35 NG/ML – or even 50 NG/ML – and some would say 75 NG/ML – is inadequate. None of the patients reviewed here – the worst eighteen per cent of the overall sample of those with definite vitamin D deficiency as defined above – had a level higher than 13 NG/ML. One easily could argue that levels not quite reaching this threshold also are worthy of attention.

As a final caveat, let me emphasize that the field of vitamin D research is moving quite rapidly. Whatever you learned several years ago probably has been superseded.

Brief Case Reports:
Male Patient #1: [censored]. The vitamin D level was ordered by his personal physician because of the patient's persistent pain. Lab results already on file 5 years earlier: [censored]. New lab results: [censored].
Female Patient #1: [censored]. The vitamin D level was ordered because she complained of hip joint pain. New lab results: [censored].
Male Patient #2: [censored]. The vitamin D level was ordered because of his noted preference for sunlight. New lab results: [censored].
Male Patient #3: [censored]. The vitamin D level was ordered because he complained vaguely of rib pain. New lab results: [censored].
Female Patient #2: [censored]. The vitamin D level was ordered

because of her persistently low calcium levels. Lab results already on file 6 months earlier: [censored]. New lab results: [censored]. Subsequent lab results 2 weeks later: [censored].

Female Patient #3: [censored]. The vitamin D level was ordered because of her joint pain. New lab results: [censored].

Female Patient #4: [censored]. The vitamin D level was ordered because of her persistent pain. New lab results: [censored].

Female Patient #5: [censored]. The vitamin D level was ordered because of her current chronic pain. New lab results: [censored].

Male Patient #4: [censored]. The vitamin D level was ordered because of his history of erratic calcium levels. New lab results: [censored].

Female Patient #6: [censored]. The vitamin D level was ordered because of her many varieties of pain. New lab results: [censored].

Male Patient #5: [censored]. The vitamin D level was ordered because of his orthopedic issues and associated pain. New lab results: [censored].

Female Patient #7: [censored]. The vitamin D level was ordered because of her global muscle pain. New lab results: [censored].

Female Patient #8: [censored]. The vitamin D level was ordered because of her persistent pain. New lab results: [censored].

Male Patient #6: [censored]. The vitamin D level was ordered because of his persistent leg pain. Lab results already on file 5 weeks earlier: [censored]. New lab results: [censored].

Male Patient #7: [censored]. The vitamin D level was ordered because of his history of frequent fractures with residual pain. New lab results: [censored].

Male Patient #8: [censored]. The vitamin D level was ordered because of his chronic low-grade lower back pain. New lab results: [censored].

Male Patient #9: [censored]. The vitamin D level was ordered because of his persistent knee pain. New lab results: [censored].

Male patient #10: [censored]. The vitamin D level was ordered because of his chronic vague leg aches. New lab results: [censored].

Male Patient #11: [censored]. The vitamin D level was ordered because of his chronic pain. New lab results: [censored]. Unfortunately, correcting vitamin D deficiency is not always easily achieved. New lab result 10 months later: [censored].

Discussion:

Of the 19 patients with severe vitamin D deficiency cited in this convenience sample, note that the vast majority had some degree of persistent pain – frequently related to bones or joints, that about a third of those had significant iron deficiency, and that about a sixth of those had calcium issues. Of the patients cited, note that only about a tenth had lab data already on file that suggested vitamin D deficiency and only about a fifth had clinical data already on file that suggested vitamin D deficiency. Almost all had self-diagnosed "depression," but most seemed uncertain that "depression" was the correct diagnosis – which is somewhat unusual for patients presenting at an outpatient psychiatric clinic.

Notice some of the words being used in these brief case histories: "moving in quick-sand" – "wasn't being responsive enough" – "an inability to do anything until I calm myself down" – "pretty withdrawn" – "takes me longer and longer to do things" – "can't sit still" – "a state of just not caring any more" – "my mind wanders off" – "I'll catch myself doing nothing" – "It's like I'm always waiting for something to happen" – "I don't feel comfortable around people". These cases were collected without any psychiatric preconceptions whatsoever, so it came as quite a surprise to note that themes about global sluggishness and vague discomfort were front and center.

None of these patients were viewed by themselves or others as severely or even moderately depressed. Furthermore, none of these patients would be considered as the ideal candidates for the clinical trial of an active pharmaceutical agent as one would have to document movement from "vague mild depression" to "no depression" – which would be hard to distinguish from a placebo response.

Medical articles focusing on severe vitamin D deficiency in otherwise healthy patients are rare. There is an apparent growing consideration, however, that some degree of vitamin D deficiency is far more ubiquitous than had been appreciated even a decade ago. While an analysis published in early 2013 correlated severity of vitamin deficiency with likelihood of suicide in active duty military personnel, a review published in early 2010 correlated some degree of vitamin D deficiency with depression in the elderly, a study published in early 2010 correlated the same with depression in those with cardiovascular disorder – especially in men over age 64 – and a study published in late 2008 correlated the same with depression in the obese, there is only one known rigorous evaluation of vitamin D and any psychologic variable in more commonplace adults. A US population study published in late 2010, of 7,970 non-institutionalized men and women between 15 and 39 years old, found that those with a serum 25()H) D level lower than 50 nmol/L were significantly more likely to be depressed than those having a level higher than 75 nmol/L [note how high this standard is]. A Swedish population study published in early 2010, of 33,000 women between 30 and 49 years old, found that, a decade later, those in the highest quartile of vitamin D intake had a 37% lower risk of having developed psychotic-like symptoms. A single-case study published in late 2010 noted rapid resolution of excessive daytime sleepiness after the correction of severe vitamin D deficiency. No one else seems to have noted the clustering of psychological concerns outlined above – global sluggishness and vague discomfort – a clustering that is very different from other varieties of apparent depression. If a patient presents with an ill-defined mild but bothersome depression-like condition AND has clear concerns about persistent pain, then one might want to consider ordering a 25-hydroxy vitamin D level.

> "National data demonstrate a marked decrease in serum 25(OH)D levels from the 1988-1994 to the 2001-2004 NHANES [US National Health & Nutrition Examination Survey] data collections."
> Adit A. Ginde, Mark C. Liu, Carlos A Camargo, Jr.

Severe vitamin D deficiency is common in locations lacking an abundance of sunlight, which helps human bodies to generate vitamin D –

but deficiency occurs even in those locations not so lacking, as some people have hours of work, manners of dress, or darkness of skin that minimize such exposure, and some people have excessive weight, which raises requirements. One could argue that all patients having one of these circumstances should have a baseline 25-hydroxy vitamin D level obtained.

As a final note, it is worth remembering that severe vitamin D deficiency – or even mild vitamin D deficiency, for that matter – may have real consequences on patients' overall well-being. Data published primarily during the last decade (following up on numerous animal studies) suggests that even mild vitamin D deficiency in otherwise healthy men and women correlates with osteoporosis, myalgia, multiple sclerosis, psoriasis, arthritis, diabetes, hypertension, pneumonia, and many cancers – conditions that were either prevented or somewhat ameliorated by optimizing vitamin D. Recent preliminary data suggests that vitamin D deficiency correlates with cognitive variables and work productivity, but those questions have only begun to be explored. Being less productive in the workplace might contribute realistically to a patient's self-diagnosis of "depression" or "anxiety" – even if, in the best of all worlds, the most optimal first presentation would not be to a psychiatrist's office. Despite the growing body of data on the global consequences of vitamin D deficiency, a North American review of 278 charts, published in early 2010, found that even once the deficiency had been identified – and regardless of the severity – only 31% of the identified patients had any follow-up during the year.

To reiterate, that a patient complains of "depression" or "anxiety" does not mean that "depression" or "anxiety" is the only – or even the primary - problem. Just as acute or chronic "anti-depressant deficiency" or "anxiolytic deficiency" may not be the whole story, vitamin D deficiency – even severe vitamin D deficiency – may not be the whole story yet an important factor to take into consideration nonetheless.

References:

Kiraly SJ, Kiraly MA, Hawe RD, Makhani N. "Vitamin d as a neuroactive substance: review." Scientific World J.2006 Jan 26:6:125-39, p.1.

McCann JC, Ames BN. "Is there convincing biological or behavioral evidence linking vitamin D deficiency to brain dysfunction?" FASEB J.2008 Apr;22(4):982-1001, p.1.

Goodman BM 3rd, Artz N, Radford B, Chen IA. "Prevalence of vitamin D deficiency in adults with sickle cell disease." J Natl Med Assoc. 2010 Apr;102(4):332-5; this article came out after the current manuscript was drafted; 25-hydroxy vitamin D <10 ng/mL was found in 60% of the 142 patients tested.

Khoraminya N, Tehrani-Doost M, Jazayeri S, Hosseini A, Djazayery A. "Therapeutic effects of vitamin D as adjunctive therapy to fluoxetine in patients with major depressive disorder." Aust N Z J Psychiatry. 2013 Mar;47(3):271-5; "...double-blind, randomized, placebo-controlled trial, 42 patients with a diagnosis of major depressive disorder based on DSM-IV criteria were randomly assigned into two groups to receive daily either 1500 IU vitamin D3 plus 20 mg fluoxetine or fluoxetine alone for 8 weeks. ... The vitamin D + fluoxetine combination was significantly better than fluoxetine alone from the fourth week of treatment. ..."

Mozaffari-Khosravi H, Nabizade L, Yassini-Ardakani SM, Hadinedoushan H, Barzegar K. "The Effect of 2 Different Single Injections of High Dose of Vitamin D on Improving the Depression in Depressed Patients With Vitamin D Deficiency: A Randomized Clinical Trial." J Clin Psychopharmacol. 2013 Jun;33(3):378-85; "...120 patients who had a Beck Depression Inventory II score of 17+ and were affected with vitamin D deficiency were randomly assigned to 3 groups of 40 [one to receive a single intramuscular dose of 150,000 IU of vitamin D, one to receive 300,000 IU, and one to receive nothing]. ... The results of the study revealed that first, the correction of vitamin D deficiency improved the depression state, and second, a single injection dose of 300,000 IU of vitamin D was safe and more effective than a 150,000-IU dose."

Polak MA, Houghton LA, Reeder AI, Harper MJ, Conner TS. "Serum 25-Hydroxyvitamin D Concentrations and Depressive Symptoms among Young Adult Men and Women." Nutrients. 2014 Oct 28;6(11):4720-30;

"... a non-clinical young adult [615] sample living in Dunedin, New Zealand. ... serum 25(OH)D was negatively associated with depression symptoms before and after adjustment. ... participants in the lowest quartile were more likely to report depressive symptoms compared with those in the highest quartile. ..."

Milaneschi Y, Hoogendijk W, Lips P, Heijboer AC, Schoevers R, van Hemert AM, Beekman AT, Smit JH, Penninx BW. "The association between low vitamin D and depressive disorders." Mol Psychiatry. 2014 Apr;19(4):444-51; "...participants (aged 18-65 years) ... with a current (N=1,102) or remitted (N=790) depressive disorder (major depressive disorder, dysthymia) defined according to DSM-IV criteria, and healthy controls (N=494). ... In currently depressed persons, 25(OH)D was inversely associated with symptom severity ... suggesting a dose-response gradient, and with risk ... of having a depressive disorders at 2-year follow-up. This large cohort study indicates that low levels of 25(OH)D were associated to the presence and severity of depressive disorder suggesting that hypovitaminosis D may represent an underlying biological vulnerability for depression. ..."

Le Goaziou MF1, Kellou N, Flori M, Perdrix C, Dupraz C, Bodier E, Souweine G. "Vitamin D supplementation for diffuse musculoskeletal pain: Results of a before-and-after study." Eur J Gen Pract. 2014 Mar;20(1):3-9; "...The aim ... was to evaluate the effects of correcting a vitamin D deficiency (≤ 50 nmol/l) on DMS [diffuse musculoskeletal] pain and quality of life in adults. ... Before vitamin D supplementation, the adult study cohort (n = 49) had an adjusted mean serum 25 (OH) D level of 23.7 nmol/l, a mean pain evaluation score of 5.07 and a mean quality of life score of 3.55. After vitamin D supplementation, the adjusted mean serum 25 (OH) D level increased to 118.8 nmol/l ..., the mean quality of life score increased to 2.8 nmol/l ... and the mean pain evaluation score decreased to 2.8 ... ."

McCarty DE, Reddy A, Keigley Q, Kim PY, Cohen S, Marino AA. "Nonspecific pain is a marker for hypovitaminosis D in patients undergoing evaluation for sleep disorders: a pilot study." Nat Sci Sleep. 2013 Mar 9;5:37-42; "...patients who admitted to the presence of chronic nonspecific musculoskeletal pain ... . The mean serum 25-hydroxyvitamin

D level was 19.8 ± 11.1, with 54% of the study population having vitamin D deficiency. ... Vitamin D deficiency was prevalent in patients with sleep disorders and chronic nonspecific musculoskeletal pain on evaluation in a sleep medicine clinic. ..."

Anglin RE, Samaan Z, Walter SD, McDonald SD. "Vitamin D deficiency and depression in adults: systematic review and meta-analysis." Br J Psychiatry. 2013 Feb;202:100-7; "... One case-control study, ten cross-sectional studies and three cohort studies with a total of 31 424 participants were analysed. Lower vitamin D levels were found in people with depression compared with controls ... and there was an increased odds ratio of depression for the lowest v. highest vitamin D categories in the cross-sectional studies ... . The cohort studies showed a significantly increased hazard ratio of depression for the lowest v. highest vitamin D categories ... ."

Bertone-Johnson ER, Powers SI, Spangler L, Brunner RL, Michael YL, Larson JC, Millen AE, Bueche MN, Salmoirago-Blotcher E, Liu S, Wassertheil-Smoller S, Ockene JK, Ockene I, Manson JE. "Vitamin D intake from foods and supplements and depressive symptoms in a diverse population of older women." Am J Clin Nutr. 2011 Oct;94(4):1104-12. "Study participants were 81,189 members of the Women's Health Initiative (WHI) Observational Study who were aged 50-79 y at baseline. Vitamin D intake at baseline was measured by food-frequency and supplement-use questionnaires. Depressive symptoms at baseline and after 3 y were assessed by using the Burnam scale and current antidepressant medication use. ... our findings support a potential inverse association of vitamin D, primarily from food sources, and depressive symptoms in postmenopausal women. ..."

Bertone-Johnson ER. "Vitamin D and the occurrence of depression: causal association or circumstantial evidence?" Nutr Rev. 2009 Aug;67(8):481-92.

Plotnikoff GA, Quigley JM. "Prevalence of severe hypovitaminosis D in patients with persistent, nonspecific musculoskeletal pain." Mayo Clin Proc. 2003 Dec;78(12):1463-70.

Leavitt SB. "Vitamin D for pain: update of research evidence." http://updates.pain-topics.org/2010/01/vitamin-d-for-pain-update-of-research.html updated 17-Jan-2010; accessed 23-Mar-2010. [this is one of the best summaries by far of the medical literature]

Umhau JC, George DT, Heaney RP, Lewis MD, Ursano RJ, Heilig M, Hibbeln JR, Schwandt ML. "Low Vitamin D Status and Suicide: A Case-Control Study of Active Duty Military Service Members." PLoS One. 2013;8(1): e51543 ; "... a prospective, nested, case-control study ... . Participants were previously deployed active duty US military personnel (2002–2008) ... . Vitamin D status was estimated by measuring 25(OH) D levels in serum samples drawn within 24 months of the suicide. Each verified suicide case (n = 495) was matched to a control (n = 495) by rank, age and sex. We calculated odds ratio of suicide associated with categorical levels (octiles) of 25(OH) D, adjusted by season of serum collection. ... More than 30% of all subjects had 25(OH)D values below 20 ng/mL. ... The lowest 25(OH)D levels are associated with an increased risk for suicide. ..."

Bischoff-Ferrari HA. "Optimal serum 25-hydroxyvitamin D levels for multiple health outcomes." Adv Exp Med Biol. 2014;810:500-25; "... evidence is summarized from different studies that evaluate threshold levels for serum 25(OH)D levels in relation to bone mineral density (BMD), lower extremity function, dental health, risk of falls, fractures, cancer prevention, incident hypertension and mortality. For all endpoints, levels in the deficient range (< 50 nmol/l; < 20 ng/ml) are associated with no benefit or adverse effects, while the most advantageous serum levels for 25(OH)D appeared to be close to 75 nmol/l (30 ng/ml). ..."

Hall LM, Kimlin MG, Aronov PA, Hammock BD, Slusser JR, Woodhouse LR, Stephensen CB. "Vitamin d intake needed to maintain target serum 25-hydroxy vitamin d concentrations in participants with low sun exposure and dark skin pigmentation is substantially higher than current recommendations." J Nutr.2010 Mar;140(3):542-50, p.1. [this article also authoritatively declares 75 NG/ML as the target 25-hydroxy vitamin D level]

Barnard K, Colón-Emeric C. "Extraskeletal effects of vitamin D in older adults: cardiovascular disease, mortality, mood, and cognition." Am J Geriatr Pharmacother. 2010 Feb;8(1):4-33.

May HT, Bair TL, Lappé DL, Anderson JL, Horne BD, Carlquist JF,

Muhlestein JB. "Association of vitamin D levels with incident depression among a general cardiovascular population." Am Heart J. 2010 Jun;159(6):1037-43; "... Among a CV population > or =50 years with no history of depression, vitD levels were shown to be associated with incident depression after vitD draw. This study strengthens the hypothesis of the association between vitD and depression"; "the associations among those age > or =65 and male sex were enhanced."

Jorde R, Sneve M, Figenschau Y, Svartberg J, Waterloo K. "Effects of vitamin D supplementation on symptoms of depression in overweight and obese subjects: randomized double blind trial." J Intern Med. 2008 Dec;264(6):599-609.

Cieslak K, Feingold J1, Antonius D, Walsh-Messinger J, Dracxler R, Rosedale M, Aujero N, Keefe D, Goetz D, Goetz R, Malaspina D. "Low Vitamin D levels predict clinical features of schizophrenia." Schizophr Res. 2014 Nov;159(2):257-260; "... Vitamin D levels in 22 well-characterized schizophrenia cases were examined with respect to symptoms, cognition, and functioning. ... The results showed that 91% (20) had deficient or insufficient Vitamin D levels, which were associated with excitement and grandiosity, social anhedonia, and poverty of speech. Sex-specific analyses showed strong associations of hypovitamintosis D to negative symptoms [reduced spontaneity, involvement, and expression] and decreased premorbid adjustment in males, and to lesser hallucinations and emotional withdrawal, but increased anti-social aggression in females. ..."

Hedelin M, Löf M, Olsson M, Lewander T, Nilsson B, Hultman CM, Weiderpass E. "Dietary intake of fish, omega-3, omega-6 polyunsaturated fatty acids and vitamin D and the prevalence of psychotic-like symptoms in a cohort of 33,000 women from the general population." BMC Psychiatry. 2010 May 26;10:38.

Cannell J J. "Vitamin D and mental health." http://www.vitamindcouncil.org/mentalIllness.shtml updated 08-Jan-2010; accessed 23-Mar-2010. [written by a widely published expert on vitamin D, this is one of the best summaries by far of the soft data]

Ganji V, Milone C, Cody MM, McCarthy F, Wang YT. "Serum vitamin D concentrations are related to depression in young adult US population:

the Third National Health and Nutrition Examination Survey." Int Arch Med. 2010 Nov 11;3(1):29.

Ginde AA, Liu MC, Camargo CA Jr. "Demographic differences and trends of vitamin D insufficiency in the US population, 1988-2004." Arch Intern Med.2009 Mar 23;169(6):626-32, p.1.

Tiangga E, Gowda A, Dent JA. "Vitamin D deficiency in psychiatric in-patients and treatment with daily supplements of calcium and ergocalciferol." Psychiatr Bull.2008;32:390-393, p. 392.

Chung M, Balk EM, Brendel M, Ip S, Lau J, Lee J, Lichtenstein A, Patel K, Raman G, Tatsioni A, Terasawa T, Trikalinos TA. "Vitamin D and calcium: a systematic review of health outcomes." evidence report no. 183. Agency for Healthcare Research and Quality. publication no. 09-E015. August, 2009. http://www.ahrq.gov/downloads/pub/evidence/pdf/vitadcal/vitadcal.pdf

Heaney RP. "Long-latency deficiency disease: insights from calcium and vitamin D." Amer J Clin Nutrition.2003 Nov;78(5):912-919.

Peiris AN, Bailey BA, Manning T, Adebonojo L. "Are 25-hydroxyvitamin D levels adequately monitored following evidence of vitamin D insufficiency in veterans?" Mil Med. 2010 Jun;175(6):453-6.

Peiris AN, Bailey BA, Guha BN, Copeland R, Manning T. "Can a model predictive of vitamin D status be developed from common laboratory tests and demographic parameters?" South Med J. 2011 Sep;104(9):636-9; "... For the 14,920 available patients, several factors including triglyceride level, race, total cholesterol, body mass index, calcium level, and number of missed appointments were significantly linked to vitamin D status. However, these variables accounted for less than 15% of the variance in vitamin D levels. While the variables correctly classified vitamin D deficiency status for 71% of patients, only 33% of those who were actually deficient were correctly identified as deficient. ... Given the failure to find a sufficiently predictive model for vitamin D deficiency, we propose that there is no substitute for laboratory testing of 25(OH)D levels. ..."

Sim JJ, Lac PT, Liu IL, Meguerditchian SO, Kumar VA, Kujubu DA, Rasgon SA. "Vitamin D deficiency and anemia: a cross-sectional study." Ann Hematol. 2010 May;89(5):447-52; "... Vitamin D deficiency was defined as <30 ng/mL and anemia was defined as a hemoglobin <11 g/dL. A total of 554 subjects were included in the analysis. Anemia was present in 49% of 25-hydroxyvitamin D-deficient subjects compared with 36% with normal 25-hydroxyvitamin D levels … ."

Barchetta I, Baroni MG, Leonetti F, De Bernardinis M, Bertoccini L, Fontana M, Mazzei E, Fraioli A, Cavallo MG. "TSH levels are associated with vitamin D status and seasonality in an adult population of euthyroid adults." Clin Exp Med. 2014 Jun 13. [Epub ahead of print]; "… we recruited 294 euthyroid adults (M/F 133/161, 48.5 ± 12.4 years). … Vitamin D deficiency was diagnosed for serum 25(OH) vitamin D <25 nmol/l. … Vitamin D deficiency was strongly associated with [hypothyroidism, ie,] higher TSH [thyroid stimulating hormone] levels … after adjusting for sex, age, and sample's season. Although vitamin D deficiency was also associated with metabolic syndrome and its components, the association between TSH levels and vitamin D status persisted also considering these confounders. …"

McCarty DE. "Resolution of hypersomnia following identification and treatment of vitamin d deficiency." J Clin Sleep Med. 2010 Dec 15;6(6):605-8; "… Mechanisms for her clinical improvement could include enhanced sleep quality due to resolution of hypovitaminosis D-associated non-inflammatory myopathy, or a possible immunomodulatory effect of vitamin D decreasing central nervous system (CNS) homeostatic sleep pressure via its effects on tumor necrosis factor-alpha (TNF-α) and/or prostaglandin D2. …"

Endnote:

For comparison with the above-cited most severe cases, please consider the following slightly less severe cases of vitamin D deficiency:

Brief Case Reports:

Male Patient #12: [censored]. The vitamin D level was ordered because of his chronic pain. Lab results already on file 21 months earlier: [censored]. New lab results: [censored].

Male Patient #13: [censored]. The vitamin D level was ordered because of his many past fractures plus continuing pain. New lab results: [censored].

Female Patient #9: [censored]. The vitamin D level was ordered because of her chronic low-grade pain. New lab results: [censored].

Female Patient #10: [censored]. The vitamin D level was ordered because of her chronic pain. New lab results: [censored].

Male Patient #14: [censored]. The vitamin D level was ordered because of his persistent pain. New lab results: [censored].

Male Patient #15: [censored]. The vitamin D level was ordered because of his fractures and pain. New lab results: [censored].

Female Patient #11: [censored]. The vitamin D level was ordered because of her multiple sources of chronic pain. New lab results: [censored].

Female Patient #12: [censored]. The vitamin D level was ordered because of her chronic pain and history of hypocalcemia. Lab results already on file 1 year earlier: [censored]. Unfortunately, correcting vitamin D deficiency is not always easily achieved. New lab results: [censored].

Female Patient #13: [censored]. The vitamin D level was ordered because of her skin condition. New lab results: [censored].

Male Patient #16: [censored]. The vitamin D level was ordered because of his chronic pain. New lab results: [censored].

Female Patient #14: [censored]. The vitamin D level was ordered because of her persistent low-grade pain. New lab results: [censored].

Male Patient #17: [censored]. The vitamin D level was ordered because of his chronic pain. New lab results: [censored]. [For some unclear reason the lab did not draw the ordered "comprehensive metabolic profile" – and there was not a previous one anywhere in the available computer database – so one cannot evaluate this patient's calcium status or hydration status.]

Female Patient #15: [censored]. The vitamin D level was ordered because of her many varieties of chronic pain. New lab results: [censored]. [The folate level was ordered because of macrocytosis in the presence of normal B6, B12, and methylmalonic acid levels. Interestingly enough, chart review 8 months later revealed that she was still macrocytotic, that the vitamin D tablets and folic acid tablets had been discontinued, plus that there was no follow-up in regard to the hyperkalemia and beginning hypometabolism.

Male Patient #18: [censored]. The vitamin D level was ordered because of his chronic pain. New lab results: [censored].

Female patient #16: [censored]. The vitamin D level was ordered because of her long-standing use of an anticonvulsant. New lab results: [censored]. [Interestingly enough, chart review 8 months later revealed that she was still macrocytotic and that she was taking (as recommended) twenty-five per cent more of her seizure medication, but that the vitamin D tablets and calcium tablets had been discontinued, even though the particular anticonvulsant she was on is known to reduce vitamin D and calcium levels.]

Male Patient #19: [censored]. The vitamin D level was ordered because of recent hypocalcemia. Lab results already on file 1 day earlier: [censored]. New lab results: [censored].

Female Patient #17: [censored]. The vitamin D level was ordered because of her multiple sclerosis. Lab results already on file 5 months earlier: [censored]. New lab results: [censored]. Getting a patient to adhere to a diet or supplement regimen on a long-term basis is not always easy. This patient did become substantially more emotionally stable.

Female Patient #18: [censored]. The vitamin D level was ordered because of her chronic pain. New lab results: [censored]. Lab results 30 months later: [censored]. Lab results 4 months after that: [censored]. Lab results 6 months after that: [censored]. Again, getting a patient to adhere to a diet or supplement regimen on a long-term basis is not always easy. Again, this patient did become substantially more emotionally stable.

Discussion:

Of this second group of 18 patients with slightly less severe vitamin D deficiency cited in this convenience sample, note that 13 – that is, 72% – had some degree of persistent pain – frequently related to bones or joints, that 2 – that is, 11% – had significant iron deficiency, and that 2 had calcium issues. Almost all had self-diagnosed "depression" or "anxiety" but, again, most seemed uncertain that either was the correct diagnosis – and, in contrast to the group of patients with more severe vitamin deficiency, almost none of this group sought further mental health services, even though their emotional symptoms were not that different.

Notice, again, some of the words being used in these brief case histories: "muscles are tight" – "drains energy" – "can't sit still" – "it's my wife's opinion that I'm depressed" – "don't want to do anything" – "not doing well" – "not able to finish anything" – "feel like 'crap'" – "situations tense me up" – "not being in a mood to put up with people". These cases, like the previous ones, were collected without any psychiatric preconceptions whatsoever, so it came as quite a surprise to note that none of these patients were viewed by themselves or others as severely or even moderately depressed – although all might view themselves as vaguely ineffective and uncomfortable. While those with the most severe vitamin D deficiency were unsure why they had come to a psychiatrist's office but they kept coming back, those with slightly less severe vitamin D deficiency were equally unsure and did not come back – but tended not to seek otherwise comprehensive health care either.

The global conclusion remains: if a patient appears to be vaguely sluggish, ineffective, and uncomfortable – but not clearly significantly depressed – AND has clear concerns about persistent pain, then one might want to consider ordering a 25-hydroxy vitamin D level. Taking into account the entire group of patients with levels lower than 20 NG/ML, 19% had significant or severe incidental iron deficiency and an astounding 79% had some variety of chronic pain. While some of these patients would have chosen to consult with a mental health professional even if their vitamin D deficiency already had been adequately treated, it is doubtful that all would have chosen that route.

V. Definite Hypercalcemia

> "*Fatigue, weakness*, mild gastrointestinal symptoms (*constipation, abdominal pain*), changes in *intellectual performance*, and *depression* may all be manifestations of hypercalcemia or excessive PTH [parathyroid hormone]."
> David M. Stovik

> "symptoms were noted not only in patients with very high serum calcium values but also in association with mild or moderate hypercalcaemia. The most common symptoms were depressive and anxiety states … ."
> Charlotte Joborn, Jerker Hetta, Mats Palmer,
> Goran Akerstrom, Sverker Ljunghall

A significant number of patients present with the erroneous psychiatric self-diagnosis of "anxiety" or "depression" or "irritability" when hypercalcemia is more likely the primary problem – with hypercalcemia defined as a serum calcium level more than 10.2 mg/dL. Recognizing this has been impeded by the general assumption that most cases of hypercalcemia are asymptomatic – or at least easily treated, in a temporizing manner, by hydration, perhaps with the addition of a bit of table salt. Even though only about 1% of the cases – usually signaled by a correlating low PTH level – represent carcinoma, calcium deposition in soft tissues – frequently the kidneys – is not entirely benign. While hypertriglyceridemia can produce a spuriously high total serum calcium level, and hypoalbuminemia can produce a spuriously low total serum calcium level, neither appeared to be an issue with the patients under study.

First let me present several of the most illustrative cases seen in an outpatient psychiatric practice over the last three years; overall, about one and one-half per cent of the newly evaluated patients were found to have hypercalcemia. Then let me discuss the relevant medical literature – of which there is surprisingly little. Finally let me suggest some possible reasons why these cases of hypercalcemia are presenting now.

Please note in the following cases that clinical data suggestive of a non-psychiatric diagnosis frequently was available in the opening "psychiatric chief complaint," the history of medical illness, or both. Likewise, lab data suggestive of a non-psychiatric diagnosis frequently was already on file but not acted upon. Please also note that something as simple as a "comprehensive metabolic profile" frequently provided sufficient information; that is, that while more "exotic" lab tests might be useful for confirmation of the diagnosis, frequently they were not really needed.

Let me emphasize that only the most severe cases have been chosen for consideration in this study. None of the patients reviewed here had a total calcium level lower than 10.6 mg/dL. One easily could argue that levels not quite reaching this threshold also are worthy of attention.

Brief Case Reports:

Female Patient #1: [censored]. Lab results already on file 5 years earlier: [censored]. This was possibly notable in that "irritability" had been a long-standing issue, and the hypercalcemia was in the context of hyperalbuminemia – that is, most likely accurate. New lab result 4.5 months later, noting mild hyperlipemia, which could raise the total calcium level: [censored]. Interestingly enough, 10 months after the last indication of hypercalcemia, she was prescribed calcium/ vitamin-D tablets because she was "in the age range for developing osteoporosis." Consequent – and most likely accurate – new lab results: [censored]. Lab results 4 months later after being asked to stop using the calcium/ vitamin D tablets: [censored]. Lab results 10 months after that, while on a low-sugar/ high-magnesium diet, with enhanced mood stability:

[censored].

Female Patient #2: [censored]. There were no previous calcium levels on file. New lab result: [censored].

Male Patient #1: [censored]. There were no previous calcium levels on file. New lab result: [censored]. He was missing one kidney and was found to have 2+ urinary protein; interestingly enough, while chart notes reveal that this was a concern to him, a renal diagnosis never ended up on the chart.

Male Patient #2: [censored]. There were no previous calcium levels on file. New lab results: [censored]. He was missing one kidney and was found to have a high urine microalbumin level; he was placed on disabiity with a renal diagnosis.

Male Patient #3: [censored]. Lab results already on file 15 months earlier: [censored]. New lab results including an ionized calcium level in the context of hyperalbuminemia: [censored].

Female Patient #3: [censored]. Lab result already on file 4 months earlier: [censored]. New lab results: [censored].

Discussion:

Of the patients with hypercalcemia cited in this convenience sample, note that not quite half had some variety of somewhat ego-alien irritability, that not quite half spoke of depression, that over a third had sleep disorder, that just under a third spoke of anxiety, that just under a third had immediate stomach nausea/ knotting/ tension upon awakening to start the day, and that just over a fifth had an immediate sense of dread/ anxiety/ fear upon awakening to start the day; muscle tightness was mentioned by several patients, while kicking, headache, and forgetfulness each were mentioned by at least one patient. To reiterate slightly, not quite a half mentioned some kind of notable symptom that would manifest immediately upon awakening to start the day. Of the patients cited, note that only several had lab data already on file that suggested hypercalcemia.

Medical articles focusing on hypercalcemia in otherwise healthy patients are rare. Published estimates of the prevalence of hypercalcemia are few and not recent but suggest that less than 1% in a general population has this problem compared to slightly more than 1% in a hospitalized sample – with the prevalence increasing with age in women but not in men. One of the most interesting articles, published in 1981, found a prevalence of 1.4% in a hospitalized sample – very similar to the prevalence found in this current sample of new outpatient psychiatric evaluations – but found that physicians investigated the finding in only 24% of the cases.

To reiterate, that a patient complains of "depression" or "anxiety" does not mean that "depression" or "anxiety" is the only – or even the primary – problem. Just as acute or chronic "anti-depressant deficiency" or "anxiolytic deficiency" may not be the whole story, hypercalcemia may not be the whole story yet an important factor to take into consideration nonetheless. While some of these patients would have chosen to consult with a mental health professional even if their hypercalcemia already had been adequately treated, it is doubtful that all would have chosen that route.

References:

Mitchell W, Feldman F. "Neuropsychiatric aspects of hypokalemia." CMAJ. 1968 Jan 06;98:49-51; p.51.

Stovik DM. "Chapter 96: approach to the patient with hypercalcemia." in Goroll AH & Mulley AG Jr. Primary Care Medicine: Office Evaluation and Management of the Adult Patient. 6th edition. Philadelphia: Wolters Kluver, 2009. p.742.

Joborn C, Hetta J, Palmer M, Akerstrom G, Ljunghall S. "Psychiatric symptomatology in patients with primary hyperparathyroidism." Ups J Med Sci.1986;91(1):77-87; p.77.

Sachmechi I, Shah G, Rezainadimi L, Blaustein DA, Rosner F. "Misleading acute hypercalcemia due to hyperlipidemia; a method dependent error." Endocr Pract.1997 Sep-Oct;3(5):293-6.

Parent X, Spielmann C, Hanser AM. ["'Corrected' calcium: calcium status underestimation in non-hypoalbuminemic patients and in hypercalcemic patients."] [Article in French] Ann Biol Clin (Paris). 2009 Jul-Aug;67(4):411-8. [while hypoalbuminemia supports the accuracy of apparent hypocalcemia, hyperalbuminemia less reliably supports the accuracy of apparent hypercalcemia]

Blind E, Raue F, Zisterer A, Kohl B, Ziegler R. ["Epidemiology of hypercalcemia. Significance of the determination of intact parathyroid hormone for differential diagnosis."] [Article in German] Dtsch Med Wochenschr. 1990 Nov 16;115(46):1739-45.

Palmér M, Jakobsson S, Akerström G, Ljunghall S. "Prevalence of hypercalcaemia in a health survey: a 14-year follow-up study of serum calcium values." Eur J Clin Invest. 1988 Feb;18(1):39-46.

Christensson T, Hellström K, Wengle B. "Hypercalcemia and primary hyperparathyroidism. Prevalence in patients receiving thiazides as detected in a health screen." Arch Intern Med. 1977 Sep;137(9):1138-42.

Finnis WA, Cohanim M, Yendt ER. "Unsuspected hypercalcemia among adults in hospital." Can Med Assoc J. 1981 Sep 15;125(6):561-4.

VI. Definite Magnesium Deficiency

"Until recently the physiological role of magnesium was essentially ignored. However, with the development of new technologies ... , there has been an explosion of interest in the molecular, biochemical, physiological and pharmacological functions of magnesium."
Rhian M. Touryz

"Although clinical deficiency was first reported in 1934 ... . Before the 1950s, textbooks of medicine, pediatrics and biochemistry did not mention magnesium disturbances."
Edmund B. Flink

"In contrast to vitamins, marginal mineral deficiencies impair performance. ... Magnesium deprivation increases oxygen requirements to complete submaximal exercise and reduces endurance performance."
Henry C. Lukaski

An impressive number of patients present with the erroneous psychiatric self-diagnosis of "depression" or "anxiety" or "irritability" when definite magnesium deficiency is more likely the primary problem – with "hypomagnesemia" defined as a serum magnesium level less than 1.7 where the "normal" range begins at 1.8 MG/DL. Recognizing this has been impeded by a continuing general assumption that since serum magnesium levels become more unreliable the higher they rise they cannot be of any use – even though articles in mid-2008 and late-2009 point out that the reverse situation is more to the point – that serum magnesium levels become more reliable the lower they are – especially if below 1.7 MG/DL. Appreciating the reality of magnesium deficiency also has been impeded by a continuing general assumption that since serum magnesium levels fluctuate with the level of hydration they cannot be of any use – even though these fluctuations tend to lead more commonly toward under-diagnosis than toward over-diagnosis. As a study published in early 1992 pointed out, when strenuous physical activity causes a serum magnesium level to rise, this suggests a reduction in exchangeable body stores, and most likely reflects the onset of actual magnesium deficiency. Articles published in 1985 and 1991, respectively, noted that simultaneous hyperalbuminemia and simultaneous hypocalcemia, when present, both tend to confirm the severity of magnesium depletion. That is, while a high magnesium level might be suspect, a low magnesium level is not to be ignored.

That magnesium tablets are extraordinarily inexpensive presents another problem. While correcting magnesium deficiency may be worth the effort in terms of medical benefit to a self-defined suffering patient, it is unlikely to be worth the effort in terms of financial benefit to a pharmaceutical company. An early 2010 article, acknowledging this financial impediment as well as the difficulty of directly confirming benefit if the patient's level is over 1.7 MG/DL, points out the sheer magnitude of articles correlating magnesium deficiency with at least 11 clinical syndromes, as well as that of articles correlating magnesium supplementation with a reduction of pathology. That is, the "hard" data supports keeping patients' serum magnesium levels above 1.7, while the "soft" data supports keeping them much higher.

Let me emphasize that only definite cases have been chosen for consideration in this study. Psychiatric skepticism regarding even a correlation – let alone any implication of causation – between magnesium deficiency and anxiety, irritability, or negativity appears to be so high that focusing on anything less than the most definite cases would be a waste of effort. While patients having a serum magnesium level of at least 1.8 MG/DL currently are defined as "normal," one could argue that any level less than 2.0 MG/DL is inadequate. Of the patients reviewed here – that is, the worst fourth of the overall sample of those with definite magnesium deficiency as defined above – about half had a level of 1.5 MG/DL and about half had a level of 1.6 MG/DL. One easily could argue that levels not quite reaching this threshold also are worthy of attention, but this study will consider only those cases for which there is minimal room for disagreement. Since many of the patients in the overall sample were begun on anti-depressant or anxiolytic medication and/ or were lost to follow-up, some emphasis will be placed on those patients for whom such prescriptions were not written and for whom there was follow-up.

Brief Case Reports:

Male Patient #1: [censored]. New lab results: [censored]. Hypoalbuminemia tends to enhance hypomagnesemia; available data are sparse, but the opposite also appears to be true: hyperalbuminemia tends to enhance hypermagnesemia – which suggests that this patient's true magnesium level must be slightly lower than that reported.

Male Patient #2: [censored]. New lab results: [censored].

Female Patient #1: [censored]. New lab results: [censored].

Female Patient #2: [censored]. New lab results: [censored]. While hypoalbuminema tends to enhance hypomagnesemia, dehydration tends to minimize hypomagnesemia – which overall suggests that this patient's true magnesium level must be slightly lower than that reported.

Female Patient #3: [censored]. New lab results: [censored].

Female Patient #4: [censored]. New lab results: [censored].

Female patient #5: [censored]. New lab results: [censored].

Female Patient #6: [censored]. New lab results: [censored]. Hypoalbuminemia tends to enhance hypomagnesemia – which suggests that this patient's true magnesium level must be slightly higher than that reported. Lab results after being on magnesium tablets twice a day for 6 months: [censored].

Male patient #3: [censored]. New lab results: [censored]. Over-hydration tends to augment apparent hypomagnesemia – which suggests that this patient's true magnesium level must be slightly higher than that reported.

Female patient #7: [censored]. New lab results: [censored]. Again, over-hydration tends to augment apparent hypomagnesemia – which suggests that this patient's true magnesium level must be slightly higher than that reported.

Female Patient #8: [censored]. New lab results: [censored].

Female Patient #9: [censored]. New lab results: [censored].

Female Patient #10: [censored]. New lab results: [censored].

Male Patient #4: [censored]. New lab results: [censored]. Dehydration tends to minimize hypomagnesemia – which suggests that this patient's true magnesium level must be slightly lower than that reported.

Male Patient #5: [censored]. New lab results: [censored].

Male Patient #6: [censored]. New lab results: [censored].

Male Patient #7: [censored]. New lab results: [censored].

Male Patient #8: [censored]. New lab results: [censored].

Male Patient #9: [censored]. New lab results: [censored]. Again, hyperalbuminemia tends to enhance hypermagnesemia – which suggests that this patient's true magnesium level must be slightly lower than that reported.

Male Patient #10: [censored]. New lab results: [censored].

Female Patient #11: [censored]. New lab results: [censored]. Again, over-hydration tends to augment apparent hypomagnesemia – which suggests that this patient's true magnesium level must be slightly higher than that reported.

Discussion:

Of the 21 patients with definite magnesium deficiency cited in this convenience sample, note that over half had an immediate sense of dread/ anxiety/ fear upon awakening to start the day, that over a third had immediate stomach nausea/ knotting/ tension upon awakening to start the day, that over a third had some variety of somewhat ego-alien irritability, that a third had nocturnal twitching/ kicking, that just under a third had some variety of over-thinking/ obsession, and that about a fifth had some difficulty with attention/ concentration. To reiterate slightly, the vast majority mentioned some kind of notable symptom that would manifest immediately upon awakening to start the day. Of the patients cited, note that none had lab data already on file that suggested magnesium deficiency – primarily because none had had a previous magnesium level drawn. Almost all had self-diagnosed either "depression" or "anxiety" but many seemed uncertain that either was the correct diagnosis. Those who had follow-up uniformly reported an almost immediate positive response to taking magnesium tablets. Many senior neurologists might recognize the above-noted symptom clusters as similar to those encountered in patients with untreated seizure disorder, but in some clinical settings obtaining neurologic consultation is close to impossible and/ or psychiatrists are not authorized to diagnose seizure disorder, even though many psychiatrists prescribe anticonvulsants daily.

> "The possible anticonvulsant activity of magnesium may be related to its role as an N-methyl-D-aspartate (NMDA) receptor antagonist … ."
> Anna G. Euser, Marilyn J. Cipolla

Of the patients cited, note that only one trended toward hypocalcemia and that only two trended toward hypercalcemia; that is, generally hypocalcemia was not skewing the electrolyte situation and hypercalcemia was not skewing the psychologic phenomena. Similarly, note that only one had definite hypoalbuminemia and that only two had definite hyperalbuminemia; that is, generally albumin levels were not skewing the magnesium level. Again similarly, note that only two had hypernatremia and that only four had hyponatremia; that is, generally hydration levels were not skewing the results. In summary, of the cited patients, very few had any potentially confounding factors that deserved consideration.

Medical articles focusing on definite magnesium deficiency in otherwise healthy patients are rare. Published estimates of the prevalence of definite magnesium deficiency vary widely – ranging from 2.5 to 15 %. Many studies suggest that the more physically ill the patient the more likely definite magnesium deficiency is present. A Japanese study of 1,246 magnesium deficient patients published in late 1990 found that the most common clinical findings were "personality changes" mimicking "depression," and that therefore differentiation from true psychiatric disorder was important. One of the more interesting – and most cited – studies, published in 1990, looked at those situations in which physicians ordered an electrolyte panel without also ordering a magnesium level – which was ninety-three per cent of the time; within this context lab personnel ran a magnesium level even if it had not been ordered and forty-seven per cent of the time the patient was found to have some degree of magnesium deficiency.

> "... detection of ... hypokalemia, hypophosphatemia, hyponatremia, or hypocalcemia ... should alert the clinician to order serum magnesium determinations because of the frequent association of hypomagnesemia with these electrolyte perturbations." "Hypomagnesemia occurred in 42% of patients with hypokalemia, 29% of patients with hypophosphatemia, 27% of patients with hyponatremia, and 22% of patients with hypocalcemia."
> Robert Whang

Those correlations were found in 1984. A British study published in early 2010 of almost 52,000 magnesium levels found that hypokalemia predicted definite hypomagnesemia [<1.4 mEq/L] 42% of the time and that albumin-adjusted hypocalcemia also predicted definite hypomagnesemia 42% of the time. [The reverse correlations were that definite hypomagnesemia predicted hypokalemia 46% of the time and albumin-adjusted hypocalcemia 38% of the time.]

Hypomagnesemia is not benign. Among other things definite magnesium deficiency correlates with lower high density cholesterol levels, higher C-reactive protein levels, lower inflammatory cytokine production, endothelial dysfunction, and insulin resistance.

To reiterate, that a patient complains of "depression" or "anxiety" does not mean that "depression" or "anxiety" is the only – or even the primary – problem. Just as acute or chronic "anti-depressant deficiency" or "anxiolytic deficiency" may not be the whole story, magnesium deficiency may not be the whole story yet an important factor to take into consideration nonetheless. While some of these patients would have chosen to consult with a mental health professional even if their magnesium deficiency already had been adequately treated, it is doubtful that all would have chosen that route.

References:

Ayuk J, Gittoes NJ. "How should hypomagnesaemia be investigated and treated?" Clin Endocrinol (Oxf). 2011 May 13; "Hypomagnesaemia is relatively common, with an estimated prevalence in the general population ranging from 2.5% to 15%. It may result from inadequate magnesium intake, increased gastrointestinal or renal loss, or redistribution from extracellular to intracellular space. Drug-induced hypomagnesaemia, particularly related to proton pump inhibitor (PPI) therapy is being increasingly recognised. Most patients with hypomagnesaemia are asymptomatic; symptomatic magnesium depletion is often associated with multiple other biochemical abnormalities, including hypokalaemia, hypocalcaemia and metabolic acidosis. Manifestations of symptomatic hypomagnesaemia most often involve neuromuscular, cardiovascular and metabolic features. ..."

Touyz RM. "Magnesium in clinical medicine." Front Biosci. 2004 May 1; 9:1278-93, p.1278.

Flink EB. "Magnesium deficiency." W V Med J. 1990 Oct; 86(10):459-63. Review, p.459.

Iseri LT, French JH. "Magnesium: nature's physiologic calcium blocker." Am Heart J. 1984 Jul;108(1):188-93.

Lukaski HC. "Vitamin and mineral status: effects on physical performance." Nutrition. 2004 Jul-Aug; 20(7-8):632-44, p.632.

Abdelmalik PA, Politzer N, Carlen PL. "Magnesium as an effective adjunct therapy for drug resistant seizures." Can J Neurol Sci. 2012 May;39(3):323-7; "... A retrospective chart review of 22 cases of drug resistant epilepsy, where a trial of empiric oral Mg supplementation (mainly in the form of Mg-oxide) was conducted. ... Oral Mg supplementation was associated with a significant decrease in the number of seizure days per month, from 15.3 ± 13.2 (mean ± SD) to 10.2 ± 12.6 at first follow up (3-6 months, p=0.021), and to 7.8 ± 10.0 seizure days/month at second follow up (6-12 months, p=0.004). Thirty-six percent had a response rate of 75% or greater at second follow-up. Two patients reported seizure freedom. Most patients were well maintained on MgO 420 mg twice a day, or in 2 cases, Mg Lactate, without significant adverse effects, the most frequent being diarrhea (4/22). ..."

Euser AG, Cipolla MJ. "Magnesium sulfate for the treatment of eclampsia: a brief review." Stroke. 2009 Apr;40(4):1169-75; "Magnesium sulfate may act as a vasodilator, with actions in the peripheral vasculature or the cerebrovasculature, to decrease peripheral vascular resistance or relieve vasoconstriction. Additionally, magnesium sulfate may also protect the blood-brain barrier and limit cerebral edema formation, or it may act through a central anticonvulsant action. [while focusing on eclampsia, this is a major and comprehensive review of the physiologic actions of magnesium].

Mansmann HC. "Consider magnesium homeostasis: II: staging of magnesium deficiencies." Pediatric Asthma, Allergy & Immunology. Winter 1993, 7(4): 211-215, p.211; see also his web publication: "Lab Diagnosis of Magnesium Deficiency." [http://barttersite.org/lab-diagnosis-of-magnesium-deficiency/ – accessed on 06-Mar-10] June 2008; this states most clearly that the clinical value of a serum magnesium level begins at 1.7 MG/DL and lower.

Novello NP, Blumstein HA. "Hypomagnesemia: differential diagnosis & workup." August 2009 [http://emedicine.medscape.com/article/767546-diagnosis accessed 06-Mar-10], which confirms the reliability of a low serum magnesium level.

Dolev E, Burstein R, Wishnitzer R, Lubin F, Chetriet A, Shefi M, Deuster PA. "Longitudinal study of magnesium status of Israeli military recruits." Magnes Trace Elem. 1991-1992; 10(5-6):420-6, p.420.

Kroll MH, Elin RJ. "Relationships between magnesium and protein concentrations in serum." Clin Chem. 1985 Feb; 31(2):244-6, p.245.

Fatemi S, Ryzen E, Flores J, Endres DB, Rude RK. "Effect of experimental human magnesium depletion on parathyroid hormone secretion and 1, 25-dihydroxyvitamin D metabolism." J Clin Endocrinol Metab. 1991 Nov; 73(5):1067-72.

Ismail Y, Ismail AA, Ismail AA. "The underestimated problem of using serum magnesium measurements to exclude magnesium deficiency in adults; a health warning is needed for 'normal' results." Clin Chem Lab Med. 2010 Mar; 48(3):323-7; emphasizes that a serum magnesium level in the "normal" range cannot be assumed to rule out magnesium deficiency, while a definitely low level must be heeded.

Hashizume N, Mori M. "An analysis of hypermagnesemia and hypomagnesemia." Jpn J Med. 1990 Jul-Aug; 29(4):368-72; out of a sample of 6,252 patients, 165 [2.6%] had serum magnesium levels less than or equal to 1.5 MG/DL – but 1,246 [19.9%] patients had levels that were somehow abnormal.

Whang R, Ryder KW. "Frequency of hypomagnesemia and hypermagnesemia. Requested vs routine." JAMA. 1990 Jun 13; 263(22):3063-4, p.3063.

Whang R. "Predictors of clinical hypomagnesemia. Hypokalemia, hypophosphatemia, hyponatremia, and hypocalcemia." Arch Intern Med. 1984 SEP;144(9):1794-6,p.1794.

Srivastava R, Bartlett WA, Kennedy IM, Hiney A, Fletcher C, Murphy MJ. "Reflex and reflective testing: efficiency and effectiveness of adding on laboratory tests." Ann Clin Biochem. 2010 May;47(Pt 3):223-7.

Kelishadi R, Ataei E, Ardalan G, Nazemian M, Tajadini M, Heshmat R, Keikha M, Motlagh ME. "Relationship of Serum Magnesium and Vitamin D Levels in a Nationally-Representative Sample of Iranian Adolescents: The CASPIAN-III Study." Int J Prev Med. 2014 Jan;5(1):99-103; "...330 students, aged range from 10 to 18 years, consisting of an equal number of individuals with and without hypovitaminosis D. ... The mean Mg level was 0.80 ± 0.23 mg/dl with lower level in the group with hypovitaminosis D than in others ... ."

Tarleton EK, Littenberg B. "Magnesium intake and depression in adults." J Am Board Fam Med. 2015 Mar-Apr;28(2):249-56 [full free article available on the web]; "... A cross-sectional, population-based data set (National Health and Nutrition Examination Survey) was used to explore the relationship of magnesium intake and depression in 8894 US adults (mean age, 46.1 years; 47.4% men) from 2007 to 2010. Using logistic regression to model the relationship between the presence of depression (Patient Health Questionnaire score ≥5) and low magnesium intake (<184 mg/day), we examined the risk ratio (RR) of magnesium intake and its 95% confidence interval. ... After adjusting for all potential confounders, the strength of the association of very low magnesium intake with depression was statistically significant (RR = 1.16; 95% CI, 1.06-1.30). ..."

Serefko A, Szopa A, Wlaź P, Nowak G, Radziwoń-Zaleska M, Skalski M, Poleszak E. "Magnesium in depression." Pharmacol Rep. 2013;65(3):547-54 [excellent review of the preclinical & clinical data; full free article available on the web]

Sugimoto J, Romani AM, Valentin-Torres AM, Luciano AA, Ramirez Kitchen CM, Funderburg N, Mesiano S, Bernstein HB. "Magnesium decreases inflammatory cytokine production: a novel innate immunomodulatory mechanism." J Immunol. 2012 Jun 15;188(12):6338-46.

Sowa-Kućma M, Szewczyk B, Sadlik K, Piekoszewski W, Trela F, Opoka W, Poleszak E, Pilc A, Nowak G. "Zinc, magnesium and NMDA receptor alterations in the hippocampus of suicide victims." J Affect Disord. 2013 Dec;151(3):924-31; "...Zinc and magnesium, the potent antagonists of the NMDA receptor complex, are involved in the pathophysiology of depression and exhibit antidepressant activity. ... there was a statistically significant decrease (by 29% and 40%) in the potency of zinc and magnesium (respectively) to inhibit [3H] MK-801 binding to NMDA receptors in the hippocampus in suicide tissue [n= 17] relative to the [sudden death] controls [n=6]. ... Furthermore, lower concentrations (-9%) of magnesium (although not of zinc) were demonstrated in suicide tissue. ..."

Yary T, Aazami S, Soleimannejad K. "Dietary intake of magnesium may modulate depression." Biol Trace Elem Res. 2013 Mar;151(3):324-9; "... a convenience sample of 402 ... students .... The mean age of the participants was 32.54 ± 6.22 years. The results of the study demonstrated an inverse relationship between magnesium intake and depressive symptoms, which persisted even after adjustments for sex, age, body mass index, monthly expenses, close friends, living on campus, smoking (current and former), education, physical activity, and marital status."

Weglicki WB. "Hypomagnesemia and inflammation: clinical and basic aspects." Annu Rev Nutr. 2012 Aug 21;32:55-71; "… Investigations of animal and cellular responses to magnesium deficiency have found evidence of complex proinflammatory pathways that may lead to greater understanding of mediators of the pathobiology in neuronal, cardiovascular, intestinal, renal, and hematological tissues. The roles of free radicals, cytokines, neuropeptides, endotoxin, endogenous antioxidants, and vascular permeability, and interventions to limit the inflammatory response associated with these parameters, are outlined in basic studies of magnesium deficiency. …"

Rosanoff A, Weaver CM, Rude RK. "Suboptimal magnesium status in the United States: are the health consequences underestimated?" Nutr Rev. 2012 Mar;70(3):153-64; "… Cellular magnesium deficit, perhaps involving TRPM [transient receptor potential melastatin] 6/7 channels, elicits calcium-activated inflammatory cascades independent of injury or pathogens. …".

Takase B, Akima T, Satomura K, Ohsuzu F, Mastui T, Ishihara M, Kurita A. "Effects of chronic sleep deprivation on autonomic activity by examining heart rate variability, plasma catecholamine, and intracellular magnesium levels." Biomed Pharmacother. 2004 Oct; 58 Suppl 1:S35-9.

Guerrero-Romero F, Rodríguez-Morán M. "Hypomagnesemia is linked to low serum HDL-cholesterol irrespective of serum glucose values." J Diabetes Complications. 2000 Sep-Oct; 14(5):272-6.

Chaudhary DP, Sharma R, Bansal DD. "Implications of magnesium deficiency in type 2 diabetes: a review." Biol Trace Elem Res. 2009 Jul 24.

Cotruvo J & Bartram J, editors. Calcium and Magnesium in Drinking-water: Public health significance. Geneva, Switzerland: World Health Organization Press, 2009; the relative paucity of human clinical data compared to epidemiological and veterinary is notable.

Sedehizadeh S, Keogh M, Wills AJ. "Reversible hypomagnesaemia-induced subacute cerebellar syndrome." Biol Trace Elem Res. 2010 Jul 7; "On MRI imaging, a transient lesion of the cerebellar nodulus was observed, which has not, to our knowledge, been previously described in isolated hypomagnesaemia."

Kazaks AG, Uriu-Adams JY, Albertson TE, Shenoy SF, Stern JS. "Effect of oral magnesium supplementation on measures of airway resistance and subjective assessment of asthma control and quality of life in men and women with mild to moderate asthma: a randomized placebo controlled trial." J Asthma. 2010 Feb;47(1):83-92; interestingly enough, significant clinical improvement was noted at 6 months even though serum magnesium levels had not changed; that is, tissue levels once again appear to be worse than worse than serum levels [see Dolev E et al, 1991-1992, noted above].

Yousef AA, Al-deeb AE. "A double-blinded randomised controlled study of the value of sequential intravenous and oral magnesium therapy in patients with chronic low back pain with a neuropathic component." Anaesthesia. 2013 Mar;68(3):260-6; "... a cohort of 80 patients with chronic low back pain with a Leeds Assessment of Neuropathic Signs and Symptoms pain scale score $\geq$ 12, who were receiving a physical therapy programme. All patients were treated with anticonvulsants, antidepressants and simple analgesics; in addition 40 patients received placebo for 6 weeks (control group), while the other 40 patients received an intravenous magnesium infusion for 2 weeks followed by oral magnesium capsules for another 4 weeks (magnesium group). ... Our findings show that a 2-week intravenous magnesium infusion followed by 4 weeks of oral magnesium supplementation can reduce pain intensity and improve lumbar spine mobility during a 6-month period in patients with refractory chronic low back pain with a neuropathic component."

James MF. "Magnesium: an emerging drug in anaesthesia." Br J Anaesth. 2009 Oct;103(4):465-7. [this excellent summary of the physiologic actions of magnesium could easily have been published in a neuropsychiatric or more general medical journal]

Abdelmalik PA, Politzer N, Carlen PL. "Magnesium as an effective adjunct therapy for drug resistant seizures." Can J Neurol Sci. 2012 May;39(3):323-7; "... For almost a century, Mg has been used as prophylaxis and treatment of seizures associated with eclampsia. ... However, because of the availability of well-studied anticonvulsant drugs,

Mg has not been tested widely in the treatment of epileptic seizures. ... A retrospective chart review of 22 cases of drug resistant epilepsy, where a trial of empiric oral Mg supplementation (mainly in the form of Mg-oxide) was conducted. ... Oral Mg supplementation was associated with a significant decrease in the number of seizure days per month, from 15.3 ± 13.2 (mean ± SD) to 10.2 ± 12.6 at first follow up (3-6 months, p=0.021), and to 7.8 ± 10.0 seizure days/month at second follow up (6-12 months, p=0.004). Thirty-six percent had a response rate of 75% or greater at second follow-up. Two patients reported seizure freedom. ..." [despite the wealth of data in non-humans, as well as the common view that magnesium is anticonvulsant, there appears to be no solid research re the stand-alone use of magnesium in stand-alone seizures]

Zou LP, Wang X, Dong CH, Chen CH, Zhao W, Zhao RY. "Three-week combination treatment with ACTH + magnesium sulfate versus ACTH monotherapy for infantile spasms: a 24-week, randomized, open-label, follow-up study in China." Clin Ther. 2010 Apr;32(4):692-700; "... Infantile spasms (IS) is an age-specific and severe epileptic encephalopathy that occurs in infancy and early childhood and is usually refractory to conventional antiepileptic drugs. Adrenocorticotropic hormone (ACTH) has been the treatment of choice for IS, but ACTH use has been associated with infection and hypertension. Magnesium ion is an N-methyl-D-aspartic acid (NMDA)-noncompetitive antagonist that might inhibit NMDA activity and has antiepileptic and neuroprotective effects. ... Thirty-eight infants were enrolled (23 male, 15 female; median age, 9.2 months; 19 patients per group). ... Of the 12 patients who were seizure free at 24 weeks in the ACTH + MgSO(4) group, 11 (91.7%) had complete recovery (normalized EEG); this rate was 7 of 10 (70.0%) in the control group. ... Personal-social neurodevelopment was significantly improved from baseline in the group that received combination treatment. ..." [despite the wealth of data in non-humans, as well as the common view that magnesium is anticonvulsant, there appears to be no solid research re the stand-alone use of magnesium in stand-alone seizures]

Lindner G, Funk GC, Leichtle AB, Fiedler GM, Schwarz C, Eleftheriadis T, Pasch A, Mohaupt MG, Exadaktylos AK, Arampatzis S. "Impact of proton pump inhibitor use on magnesium homoeostasis: a cross-sectional study in a tertiary emergency department." Int J Clin Pract. 2014 Nov;68(11):1352-7; "... A cross-sectional study was performed in 5118 patients who had measurements of serum magnesium taken on admission to a large tertiary care ED ... . Use of PPIs predisposes patients to hypomagnesaemia [< 0.75 mmol/l {~1.8 mg/dL}] and ... to prolonged hospitalisation irrespective of the underlying morbidity, posing a critical concern.

National Academy of Sciences (U.S.) (the Committee on Mineral Requirements for Cognitive and Physical Performance of Military Personnel, the Committee on Military Nutrition Research, and the Food and Nutrition Board). Mineral Requirements for Military Personnel: Levels Needed for Cognitive and Physical Performance during Garrison Training. Washington, D.C.: National Academies Press, 2006. [This is an excellent review of what is known – and not known – about the roles of calcium, copper, iron, magnesium, selenium, and zinc in human nutrition.]

VII. Cobalamin (B-12) Deficiency

"… use of a low serum vitamin B_{12} level as the sole means of diagnosis may miss up to one half of patients with actual tissue B_{12} deficiency. … the rate of missed diagnosis … [ranges] from 10 to 26 percent when diagnosis is based on low serum vitamin B_{12} levels alone. … Elevated levels of methylmalonic acid and homocysteine are a much more sensitive diagnostic clue than a low serum B_{12} level in the diagnosis of vitamin B_{12} deficiency."
Robert C. Oh, David L. Brown

"Psychiatric manifestations can occur in the presence of low serum B12 levels but in the absence of the other well recognized neurological and hematological abnormalities of pernicious anemia. Mental or psychological changes may precede hematological signs by months or years. They can be the initial symptoms or the only ones."
Curtiss J. Durand, Sophie Mary, Perrrine Brazo,
Sonja Dollfus

A significant number of patients present with the erroneous psychiatric self-diagnosis of "anxiety" or "depression" when cobalamin deficiency is more likely the primary problem. Recognizing this has been impeded by a continuing general assumption that serum vitamin B-12 levels – more properly called "cobalamin levels" – are unreliable; while there may be some truth to this it misses the point – that serum "methylmalonic acid" levels as a proxy are considered quite reliable. Appreciating the reality of cobalamin deficiency also has been impeded by a past association of "B-12 shots" rightly or wrongly with quackery. With the advent of higher oral doses and of sublingual doses there has been less derogation of such treatment. While a high serum folate level can artificially raise the serum cobalamin level, this would not be an issue with the patients under study. Also, while correcting cobalamin deficiency may be worth the effort in terms of medical benefit to a self-defined suffering patient, it is unlikely to be worth the effort in terms of financial benefit to a pharmaceutical company. [In recent years cobalamin injections have been considered appropriate for use with the most severely deficient patients but financial profit potential is minimal.]

First let me present several of the most illustrative cases seen in an outpatient psychiatric practice over the last three years; overall, about 3.5 per cent of the newly evaluated patients were found to have cobalamin deficiency. Then let me discuss the relevant medical literature – of which there is surprisingly little. Finally let me suggest some possible reasons why these cases of cobalamin deficiency are presenting now.

Please note in the following cases that lab data suggestive of a non-psychiatric diagnosis frequently was already on file but not acted upon. Please also note that something as simple as a "complete blood count" in conjunction with a "comprehensive metabolic profile" frequently provided sufficient information; that is, that while a more "exotic" lab test – a methylmalonic acid (MMA) level – might be useful for confirmation of the diagnosis, frequently one could deduce it – by the rarity of folate deficiency and the presence of macrocytosis coupled with the absence of a low aspartate aminotransferase (AST) level [previously known as a serum glutamic-oxaloacetic transaminase (SGOT) level]; in the presence of a low AST level, pyridoxine (B-6) deficiency would have been a consideration.

Let me emphasize that only definite cases – that is, those that have elevated MMA levels – have been chosen for consideration in this study. While common sense might suggest ordering a "vitamin B-12" level then noting if it was low – and that can be done – a high MMA level turns out to be a more accurate and earlier indication of cobalamin deficiency in tissues; currently both levels frequently are ordered, although an MMA would suffice. With the following cases, frequently the "complete blood count" and "comprehensive metabolic profile" results had come back while the patient was still in the clinic building – so that it was not that difficult to have the patient called back to the lab for a MMA level. [During the time span of this study, with this population, cobalamin deficiency was confirmed about six times more frequently and pyridoxine deficiency about thirty times more frequently than was folate deficiency, so macrocytosis in the absence of a low AST almost always signaled cobalamin deficiency.]

Brief Case Reports:

With patients who are post-gastric bypass, one expects to find several simultaneous vitamin and mineral deficiencies, but generally one does not encounter this otherwise. In the space of 1 year 8 patients were found to have a high methylmalonic acid level, and all 8 were found to have at least one other vitamin or mineral deficiency.

Female Patient #1: [censored]. The methylmalonic acid level was ordered because of her restlessness in the middle of the night and because of current hypotheses relating to cardiomyopathy. New lab results: [censored].

Female Patient #2: [censored]. The methylmalonic acid level was ordered because of her earlier macrocytosis. Lab results already on file 9 weeks earlier: [censored]. New lab results: [censored].

Female Patient #3: [censored]. The methylmalonic acid level was ordered because of her earlier macrocytosis. Lab results already on file 6 weeks earlier: [censored]. New lab results: [censored].

Female Patient #4: [censored]. The methylmalonic acid level was ordered because of her earlier macrocytosis. Lab results already on file 6.5 months earlier: [censored]. New lab results: [censored].

Male Patient #1: [censored]. The methylmalonic acid level was ordered because of his earlier macrocytosis. Lab results already on file 2.5 months earlier: [censored]. New lab results: [censored]. New lab result 2 days later: [censored].

Male Patient #2: [censored]. The methylmalonic acid level was ordered because of his earlier macrocytosis and middling vitamin B12 level. Lab results already on file 9 months earlier: [censored]. New lab results: [censored].

Female Patient #5: [censored]. The methylmalonic acid level was ordered because of her earlier severe microcytosis apparently unresponsive to iron in the context of a normal protein electrophoresis. Lab results on file 3 months earlier: [censored]. New lab results: [censored].

Female Patient #6: [censored]. New lab results: [censored]. The methylmalonic acid level was ordered because of a question of macrocytosis. Lab results 3 weeks later: [censored].

Discussion:

Of the 8 patients with definite B12 deficiency cited in this convenience sample, note that 5 had self-diagnosed some mixture of anxiety/ tension and that 3 had self-diagnosed some mixture of depression/ moodiness. Also note that of the 8 patients cited, 2 had definite and 1 had almost B6 deficiency, 2 had hyponatremia, 1 had hypophosphatemia, 1 had iron deficiency, 1 had zinc deficiency, 1 had hypocalcemia, 1 had hypercalcemia, and 1 had hypomagnesemia. None of the 8 patients cited had simple, uncomplicated depression or anxiety and none had simple, uncomplicated B12 deficiency.

Medical articles focusing on cobalamin deficiency in otherwise healthy patients are rare. A study published in 1998 of over 11,000 non-ill children and adults estimated a 3% incidence of cobalamin deficiency in the United States. Another study published in early 2010, of 3,503 older North Americans, found that for every additional 10mcg of cobalamin consumed over an average of 7 years there was a 2% drop in the incidence of depression per year.

So why are so many patients suddenly presenting with the erroneous psychiatric self-diagnosis of "anxiety" or "depression" when cobalamin deficiency is more likely the primary problem? Let me discuss several possibilities. Some of the sparse literature suggests the role of excessive intake of either alcohol or caffeine, but this factor was present in only 2 of the above-cited 8 cases, and 2 of the above-cited 8 cases used neither alcohol nor caffeine at all.

Cobalamin deficiency also has been cited as correlating with pyridoxine deficiency, but their comparative frequencies vary widely according to the population studied. With the specific outpatient sample currently under study, cases of definite pyridoxine deficiency were 5 times more common than those of definite cobalamin deficiency.

Proton pump inhibitors, used for the treatment of gastroesophageal reflux, have emerged as a major cause of reduced cobalamin absorption – as well as of associated calcium, iron, magnesium, and vitamin C deficiencies. While the long-term use proton pump inhibitors has become somewhat ubiquitous, the exact prevalence of their use in the current patient sample is not known.

Numerous articles discuss the role of cobalamin deficiency in geriatric cognitive disorders, but few concern younger patients. One study published in early 2010 found that for school children in India, aged 6 to 10, cobalamin deficiency correlated with reduced recall and short-term memory. An older but especially disturbing study published in 1988 found that while macrocytosis is generally considered a hallmark of cobalamin deficiency it was present only 72 per cent of the time in patients having coexisting cobalamin deficiency and neuropsychiatric symptoms.

To reiterate, that a patient complains of "depression" or "anxiety" does not mean that "depression" or "anxiety" is the only – or even the primary – problem. Just as acute or chronic "anti-depressant deficiency" or "anxiolytic deficiency" may not be the whole story, cobalamin deficiency may not be the whole story yet an important factor to take into consideration nonetheless. While some of these patients would have chosen to consult with a mental health professional even if their cobalamin deficiency already had been adequately treated, it is doubtful that all would have chosen that route.

References:

Mitchell W, Feldman F. "Neuropsychiatric aspects of hypokalemia." CMAJ. 1968 Jan 06;98:49-51; p.51.

Oh R C, Brown DL. "Vitamin B12 deficiency." Am Fam Physician. 2003 Mar 1;67(5):979-986.

Sharma V1, Biswas D. "Cobalamin deficiency presenting as obsessive compulsive disorder: case report." Gen Hosp Psychiatry. 2012 Sep-Oct;34(5):578; "... We report a case of middle-aged man presenting with OCD, low serum cobalamin and a positive family history of vitamin B12 deficiency who responded well to methylcobalamin replacement.

Tufan AE, Bilici R, Usta G, Erdoğan A. "Mood disorder with mixed, psychotic features due to vitamin b12 deficiency in an adolescent: case report." Child Adolesc Psychiatry Ment Health. 2012 Jun 22;6(1):25; "...a 16-year old, male adolescent who presented with mixed mood disorder symptoms with psychotic features. Chief complaints were 'irritability, regressive behavior, apathy, crying and truancy' which lasted for a year. ... [He] had started to display anxiety during separation from his mother, wept frequently and complained of vague pains, lethargy, forgetfulness and reduced concentration alternating with racing thoughts, irritability, anhedonia, distractibility, reduced sleep and appetite. Speech was reduced and he became progressively isolated from his peers. ... [He] was frequently agitated, spent his free time in front of his computer and ... ran excessive debts ... buying items on-line. Premorbid personality was unremarkable with no substance use/ exposure or infections. No stressors were present. The patient was not vegetarian. Past medical history and family history was normal. Neurological examination revealed glossitis, ataxia, rigidity in both shoulders, cog-wheel rigidity in the left elbow, bilateral problems of coordination in cerebellar examination, reduced swinging of the arms and masked face. Romberg's sign was present. [notable response within 1 week to B12 injections] ... mood disorders with psychotic features especially with accompanying extrapyramidal symptoms lacking a clear etiology may be rare manifestation of vitamin B12 and/or folate deficiency ... ."

Dogan M, Ozdemir O, Sal EA, Dogan SZ, Ozdemir P, Cesur Y, Caksen H. "Psychotic disorder and extrapyramidal symptoms associated with vitamin B12 and folate deficiency." J Trop Pediatr. 2009 Jun;55(3):205-7; "... presentation of vitamin B12 deficiency-psychotic disorder, extrapyramidal symptoms in a 12-year-old boy. His symptoms responded to parenteral vitamin B12 therapy. ...

Durand C, Mary S, Brazo P, Dollfus S. ["Psychiatric manifestations of vitamin B12 deficiency: a case report"] [Article in French] Encephale. 2003 Nov-Dec;29(6):560-5; p.560.

Snow CF. "Laboratory diagnosis of vitamin B12 and folate deficiency: a guide for the primary care physician." Arch Int Med.1999 Jun 28;159(12):1289-98; p.1293.

Stabler SP. "Clinical Practice: Vitamin B12 Deficiency." N Engl J Med.2013 Jan 10;368:149-160 [excellent review, reiterating that a "serum vitamin B12 level" is grossly unreliable while an "elevated level of methylmalonic acid is reasonably specific for vitamin B12 deficiency"]

Herrmann W, Obeid R. "Cobalamin deficiency." Subcell Biochem. 2012;56:301-22; "... No single parameter can be used to diagnose cobalamin deficiency. Total serum cobalamin is neither sensitive nor it is specific for cobalamin deficiency. ... Concentrations of MMA [methylmalonic acid] and tHcy [homocysteine] increase in blood of cobalamin deficient subjects. Despite limitations of these markers in patients with renal dysfunction, concentrations of MMA and tHcy are useful functional markers of cobalamin status. The combined use of holoTC and MMA assays may better indicate cobalamin status than either of them. ..."

Selhub J, Morris MS, Jacques PF, Rosenberg IH. "Folate-vitamin B-12 interaction in relation to cognitive impairment, anemia, and biochemical indicators of vitamin B-12 deficiency." Am J Clin Nutr. 2009 Feb;89(2):702S-6S, p.702S [re that high folate intake can push B12 higher]

Wright JD, Bialostosky K, Gunter EW, Carroll MD. Najjar MF, Bowman BA, Johnson CI. "Blood folate and vitamin B12: United States, 1988-94." Vital Health Stat 11. 1998; (243):1-78.

Skarupski KA, Tangney C, Li H, Ouyang B, Evans DA, Morris MC.

"Longitudinal association of vitamin B-6, folate, and vitamin B-12 with depressive symptoms among older adults over time." Am J Clin Nutr. 2010 Aug;92(2):330-5; "… 3503 adults … . each 10 additional milligrams of vitamin B-6 and 10 additional micrograms of vitamin B-12 were associated with 2% lower odds of depressive symptoms per year. …"

Lam JR, Schneider JL, Zhao W, Corley DA. "Proton pump inhibitor and histamine 2 receptor antagonist use and vitamin B12 deficiency." JAMA. 2013 Dec 11;310(22):2435-42; "… We compared 25,956 patients having incident diagnoses of vitamin B12 deficiency between January 1997 and June 2011 with 184,199 patients without B12 deficiency. … Doses more than 1.5 PPI pills/d were more strongly associated with vitamin B12 deficiency … than were doses less than 0.75 pills/d … .Previous and current gastric acid inhibitor use was significantly associated with the presence of vitamin B12 deficiency."

McColl KE. "Effect of proton pump inhibitors on vitamins and iron." Am J Gastroenterol. 2009 Mar;104 Suppl 2:S5-9 [re malabsorption of iron, vitamin C, and cobalamin].

DeVault KR, Talley NJ. "Insights into the future of gastric acid suppression." Nat Rev Gastroenterol Hepatol. 2009 Sep;6(9):524-32 [re malabsorption of calcium, iron, and cobalamin].

Eilander A, Muthayya S, van der Knaap H, Srinivasan K, Thomas T, Kok FJ, Kurpad AV, Osendarp SJ. "Undernutrition, fatty acid and micronutrient status in relation to cognitive performance in Indian school children: a cross-sectional study." Br J Nutr. 2010 Apr;103(7):1056-64.

Lindebaum J, Healton EB, Savage DG, Brust JCM, Garrett TJ, Podell ER, Margell PD, Stabler SP, Allen RH. "Neuropsychiatric disorders caused by cobalamin deficiency in the absence of anemia or macrocytosis." N Engl J Med 1988; 318:1720-1728June 30, 1988

VIII. Definite Hypocalcemia

> "Neuronal Hyperexcitability Syndrome (NHS) is … difficult to diagnose … . With slightly varying symptoms the syndrome has also been defined as Spasmophilia and Hyperventilation Syndrome."
> Silvia Cristina, Giorgio Sandrini, Luigi Ruiz, Annalisa Verri, Massimo Musicco, Giuseppe Nappi

> "… the symptoms grouped under the label "spasmophilia" have been differently evaluated … by psychiatrists, who ascribe them to … anxiety, and by endocrinologists … for whom they are all due to neuromuscular hyperexcitability, the cause of which must be sought in the biochemistry of calcium."
> Mario Horenstein

A fair number of patients present with the erroneous psychiatric self-diagnosis of "anxiety" or "depression" – or even "Alzheimer's" – when definite hypocalcemia is more likely the primary problem – with definite hypocalcemia defined as a serum calcium level lower than 8.4 mg/dL. Recognizing this has been impeded by the general assumption that calcium-fortified foods and calcium tablets are so ubiquitous that no one possibly could consume too little – fully ignoring that consuming, absorbing, and retaining calcium are very different things. Appreciating the reality of definite hypocalcemia [as well of definite hypercalcemia] also has been impeded by the frequency of slight hypocalcemia [as well of slight hypercalcemia] – especially as the definition of what constitutes an appropriate calcium range has changed several times – generally upward – over the last decade. While hypotriglyceridemia can produce a spuriously low total serum calcium level, and hyperalbuminemia can produce a spuriously high total serum calcium level, neither appeared to be an issue with the patients under study.

Only a few of the newly evaluated patients were found to have hypocalcemia. Please note in the following cases that clinical data suggestive of a non-psychiatric diagnosis frequently was available in the opening "psychiatric chief complaint". Likewise, lab data suggestive of a non-psychiatric diagnosis frequently was already on file but not acted upon. Please also note that something as simple as a "comprehensive metabolic profile" frequently provided sufficient information; that is, that while more "exotic" lab tests – a parathyroid hormone (PTH) level and an ionized calcium level – might be useful for confirmation of the diagnosis, frequently they were not really needed.

Let me emphasize that only the most severe cases have been chosen for consideration in this study. None of the patients reviewed here had a total calcium level higher than 8.3 mg/dL. One easily could argue that levels just above this threshold also are worthy of attention.

Brief Case Reports:
    Female patient #1: [censored]. New lab results: [censored]. Lab results 3 months later: [censored]. While neither the sodium nor the albumin level is low enough to skew the calcium level downward, the moderate hyperlipemia is relevant as that would tend to skew the calcium level upward; that is, while this is not hypoparathyroidism it is definite hypocalcemia.
    Male patient #1: [censored]. Lab results already on file 8 months earlier: [censored]. New lab results: [censored]. Lab results 23 months later; [censored]. In other words, almost 2 years later he still had the same complaints and still had not yet been convinced that correcting hypocalcemia – and vitamin D deficiency – might be at least as important as seeking prescription medications for chest pain and tightness.
    Female #2: [censored]. New lab results: [censored]. Labs one year later:

[censored]. In other words, one cannot assume that correcting hypocalcemia will be instantaneous.

Female #3: [censored]. Lab results already on file 1 month earlier: [censored]. New lab results: [censored]. In other words, she had been hovering near hyponatremia and hypocalcemia – which do tend to go "hand in hand" – for quite some time; correcting either or both of these very likely would help to relieve her headaches.

Male patient #2: [censored]. Lab results already on file 1 month earlier: [censored]. New lab results [now on vitamin D]: [censored]. Upon increasing the calcium/ vitamin-D tablets – along with correction of the hypoalbuminemia – his cognition cleared.

Female patient #4: [censored]. Lab results already on file 20 months earlier: [censored]. Lab results already on file 12 months earlier: [censored]. Lab results already on file 10 months earlier: [censored]. New labs: [censored]. In other words, there was a long track record of increasing hypocalcemia.

Female patient #5: [censored]. Lab results already on file 7 months earlier: [censored]. Lab results already on record 1 month earlier: [censored]. New lab results: [censored]. Once again, there was a long track record of increasing hypocalcemia – this time with gross vitamin D deficiency.

Female patient #6: [censored]. New lab results: [censored]. Lab results 2 months later [on calcium/ vitamin-D]; [censored]. While the hypoalbuminemia would tend to skew the calcium level downward, the moderate hyperlipemia would tend to skew the calcium level upward; that is, while this is not hypoparathyroidism it is probable hypocalcemia.

Male patient #3: [censored]. New lab results: [censored]. Lab results 1 year later [on calcium/ vitamin-D]: [censored].

Female patient #7: [censored]. Lab results already on file 18 months earlier: [censored]. New lab results: [censored]. While the low triglyceride level might tend to skew the calcium level downward, this is probable hypocalcemia. The patient was lost to follow-up.

Male patient #4: [censored]. New lab results: [censored].

Female patient #8: [censored]. New lab results: [censored]. While the low albumin level might tend to skew the calcium level downward, this is probable hypocalcemia. The patient was lost to follow-up.

Discussion:

One thing that stands out immediately in this study is the older age of the patients as compared with those having other micronutrient abnormalities. In this population those with definite hypocalcemia averaged 41 years of age [similarly, those with hypercalcemia averaged 37 years of age].

Of the 12 patients with definite hypocalcemia cited in this convenience sample, note that three quarters had self-diagnosed anxiety and that over half had self-diagnosed depression. Also note that of the 12 patients cited, one third complained of memory loss. None of the 12 patients cited had simple, uncomplicated anxiety or depression or memory loss – as issues of pain, numbness, and tingling were tossed in – and none had simple, uncomplicated hypocalcemia – as deficiencies of albumin, creatinine, sodium, magnesium, and vitamin D also peppered the histories.

Medical articles focusing on definite hypocalcemia in otherwise healthy patients are rare – and generally complex – as those patients with more circumscribed magnesium, vitamin D, or parathyroid issues are easier to describe. Because of the body's various efforts toward maintaining homeostasis, definite hypocalcemia can be associated with both low [common] and very high [rare] magnesium levels – as well as with both low [common] and very high [rare] vitamin D levels – as well as with both very low [rare] and high [common] PTH levels. Frequently it is difficult to sort out which is the primary problem and which is a compensatory reaction. Compared to articles about other macronutrients, those on hypocalcemia generally have avoided offering any comments about prevalence.

To reiterate, that a patient complains of "depression" or "anxiety" does not mean that "depression" or "anxiety" is the only – or even the primary – problem. Just as acute or chronic "anti-depressant deficiency" or "anxiolytic deficiency" may not be the whole story, definite hypocalcemia may not be the whole story yet an important factor to take into consideration nonetheless. While some of these patients would have chosen to consult with a mental health professional even if their definite hypocalcemia already had been adequately treated, it is doubtful that all would have chosen that route.

> "abnormal diagnostic behavior ... leads to abnormal illness behavior ... and ... invariably [is] compounded by abnormal treatment behavior."
> Mark Awerbuch

References:

Mitchell W, Feldman F. "Neuropsychiatric aspects of hypokalemia." CMAJ. 1968 Jan 06;98:49-51; p.51.

Juan D. "Hypocalcemia. Differential diagnosis and mechanisms." Arch Intern Med. 1979 Oct;139(10):1166-71; "... mental changes (weakness, fatigue, irritability, memory loss, confusion, delusion, hallucination) ...."

Fukuyama Y, Hayashi M. "Sleep electroencephalograms and sleep stages in hypoparathyroidism." Eur Neurol. 1979;18(1):38-48.

Lawlor BA. "Hypocalcemia, hypoparathyroidism, and organic anxiety syndrome." J Clin Psychiatry. 1988 Aug;49(8):317-8.

Ang AW, Ko SM, Tan CH. "Calcium, magnesium, and psychotic symptoms in a girl with idiopathic hypoparathyroidism." Psychosom Med. 1995 May-Jun;57(3):299-302.

Thys-Jacobs S. "Micronutrients and the premenstrual syndrome: the case for calcium." J Am Coll Nutr. 2000 Apr;19(2):220-7.

Nora DB, Fricke D, Becker J, Gomes I. "Hypocalcemic myopathy without tetany due to idiopathic hypoparathyroidism: case report." Arq Neuropsiquiatr. 2004 Mar;62(1):154-7.

Bohrer T, Krannich JH. "Depression as a manifestation of latent chronic hypoparathyroidism." World J Biol Psychiatry. 2007;8(1):56-9.

Awerbuch, M. "Repetitive strain injury (RSI) or 'Kangaroo paw'." Med J Aust. 1985;142:237-238; quoted in De Lemos AI "Psychosomatic diagnosis: a literature review." Neurol Clin Neurophysiol [formerly, J Contemp Neurol]; 2000 July 14.

Conclusion:

> "if no randomized trial has been carried out for our
> patient's predicament, we must follow the trail to the
> next best external evidence and work from there."
> David L. Sackett, William M.C. Rosenberg,
> J.A. Muir Gray, R. Brian Haynes & W. Scott Richardson

Over the last 20 years many patients have been taught by their social environment not to anticipate that a physician might order specific lab tests as an intelligent response to the clinical history and presentation. The brief case summaries recorded above suggest that some physicians have forgotten to consider ordering well-chosen lab tests, have forgotten to consult the lab results already on file, and, oddly enough, have forgotten to study the results of lab tests just ordered. As the adage goes, "A stitch in time saves nine." A little more judiciously and persistently applied medical curiosity might well enhance healthcare efficiency and begin reducing the temptation for a patient to make his or her own erroneous self-diagnosis.

> "There are no shortcuts or time-sparing techniques
> to doing the right thing."
> Beau Batton

References:
   Sackett DL, Rosenberg WM, Gray JA, Haynes RB, Richardson WS. "Evidence based medicine: what it is and what it isn't." Brit Med J. 1996 Jan 13;312(7023):71-2, p.72.
   Batton B. "Healing hearts." JAMA. 2010 Sep 22/29; 304(12):1303-4, p.1303.   #

Afterword:

The censored case histories have been included toward indicating that there was a wealth of data behind this study. This whole investigation began by accident. Initially I was just collecting "teaching cases" for use with medical students – cases of non-psychiatric illness masquerading as psychiatric illness. It turned out that one out of every three new patients interviewed with the medical students had a hitherto undiagnosed non-psychiatric illness. Cases of carcinoma and endocrine disorder also were part of the mix, but the above-noted vitamin and mineral abnormalities were by far the most notable.

After discussing one of these cases with the medical students who had participated in the interview, the case report would be tossed into a locked file, without any further thought. One day, however, time became available for taking a look at the contents of that locked file. The 292 "teaching cases" (out of ~750 new evaluations) were sorted by non-psychiatric diagnosis – and thus began the organization and drafting of this manuscript. The most aberrant half of the cases was chosen for further study – primarily by correlation of the patients' initial complaints with the available lab results.

There were not any specific presuppositions about what might be found. Certainly the findings about zinc deficiency were a surprise – as were the findings about how severe vitamin D deficiency differs from only slight but definite vitamin D deficiency. To the best of my knowledge, these findings have not been reported elsewhere in the medical literature.

Clearly these findings are not statistically sound – but they are suggestive of certain cause and effect relationships – and of what productive lines of research might be pursued. These findings also are suggestive of significant problems in the non-psychiatric medical clinics associated with this particular psychiatric clinic. As noted, the owner of the facility did not seem to want to know the magnitude of the problem or even that it existed. One has to suspect that similar problems might be present at other facilities.

#

Also by
Robert Charles Powell

Available through
Amazon, Kindle, and
other fine booksellers

PENTOXIFYLLINE
:
A VERSATILE
OFF-PATENT MEDICINE
BEST NOT OVERLOOKED
:
*Overview with
Extensive Bibliography*

FREUDIAN
CONCEPTS IN
AMERICA
:
THE ROLE OF
PSYCHICAL RESEARCH IN
PREPARING THE WAY
:
1904-1934

WHEN DEATH
IS NOT
THEORETICAL
:
*The Readiness of the
Music Group 'Queen' for
Living with Freddie
Mercury's Dying*